Review Questions for

The USMLE Step 3 Examination

Review Questions for
The USMLE Step 3 Examination

Arshad Majid, MD

Department of Neurology

Hospital of the University of Pennsylvania

Review Questions Series

Series Editor: Thomas R. Gest, PhD

University of Arkansas for Medical Sciences

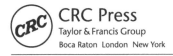

CRC Press

Taylor & Francis Group

Boca Raton London New York

CRC Press is an imprint of the
Taylor & Francis Group, an **informa** business

Published in the USA by
The Parthenon Publishing Group Inc.
One Blue Hill Plaza
PO Box 1564, Pearl River
New York 10965, USA

Published in the UK and Europe by
The Parthenon Publishing Group Limited
Casterton Hall, Carnforth
Lancs LA6 2LA, UK

Library of Congress Cataloging-in-Publication Data

Majid, Arshad.
    Review questions for the USMLE step 3 examination / Arshad Majid.
        p. cm. -- (Review questions series)
    Includes bibliographical references.
    ISBN 1-85070-063-X
    1. Physicians--Licenses--United States--Examinations--Study guides. 2.
    Medicine--Examinations, questions, etc. I. Title. II. Series.

    R834.5 .M34 2001
    616'.0076--dc21

                                                                          00-064941

British Library Cataloguing in Publication Data

Majid, Arshad
    Review questions for the USMLE Step 3 examination. –
    (Review questions series)
    1.Medicine – Examinations, questions, etc.
I.Title
610.7'6

ISBN 1-85070-063-X

CONTENTS

CONTRIBUTORS

Robert Bart, MD
Department of Pediatrics
Washington University School of Medicine
St. Louis, MO

Gabriel De Erausquin, MD, PhD
Department of Psychiatry
Washington University School of Medicine
St. Louis, MO

David Etzioni, MD
Department of Surgery
UCLA Medical Center
Los Angeles, CA

Franziska Jovin, MD
Department of Internal Medicine
Graduate Hospital
Philadelphia, PA

Jonathan Kantor, MD, MA
Department of Epidemiology and Biostatistics
Hospital of the University of Pennsylvania
Philadelphia, PA

Arshad Majid, MD
Department of Neurology
Hospital of the University of Pennsylvania
Philadelphia, PA

Shakeel Shareef, MD
Department of Ophthalmology
Geisinger Medical Center
Danville, PA

ACKNOWLEDGEMENTS

I am indebted to my parents for everything that they have done, and for their never-ending support and love.

I would like to thank the contributing editors for their excellent contributions to this book. In addition, I would like to extend my gratitude to Parthenon Publishing, particularly Meredith Ross and Nat Russo.

Finally, I thank my partner in life, Sidrah, for her help, guidance, patience and love.

Arshad Majid, MD

PREFACE

The United States Medical Licensing Examination (USMLE) Step 3 is the final step of the USMLE examination series. Passing the USMLE Step 3 is a requirement for licensure in all states. The focus of the Step 3 examination is on the clinical sciences, physical examination, data interpretation and appropriate management in different clinical settings. Parthenon's USMLE Step 3 review contains 'high yield' questions carefully written to cover the material typically encountered in the actual exam, allowing you to identify areas that need greater focus in your preparation. In addition, like the actual exam, this review book contains high quality color plates in a special section of the book. Explanations for all questions including references are given.

We believe that this review will prove to be an invaluable resource for physicians preparing for the last USMLE hurdle.

INTRODUCTION

The purpose of the USMLE Step 3 examination

According to the USMLE board, the purpose of the Step 3 examination is to determine whether a physician possesses the medical knowledge and understanding of clinical science for unsupervised practice of medicine in the United States. There is special emphasis on patient management in ambulatory care settings.

The emphasis of the Step 3 is on physician tasks, namely, evaluating severity of patient problems and managing therapy. Assessment of clinical judgement will be a prominent feature of this examination. Clinical problems involve common, mainstream, high impact diseases. Less common but important clinical problems are also tested. The questions are predominantly patient-centered, beginning with a description of a clinical encounter (vignette). The test questions pose challenges that require clinical decisions or judgement. There is special emphasis on ambulatory patient encounters. Inpatient encounters of significant acuity and complexity are also examined. Provision is made in the examination for testing applied basic science concepts, especially as they relate to prognosis or management.

Examination format

The Step 3 examination consists of multiple-choice questions, some in conjunction with pictorial material.

The Step 3 examination is a 2-day examination consisting of four tests of multiple-choice items. Each test contains approximately 180 questions. You will take two tests of the examination on the first day and two tests on the second day. You will be allowed 3 hours and 15 minutes to complete each test.

The standard, one best choice format is used. Questions are grouped in each test book according to the clinical setting. The questions may be supplemented by photographs. Assessing the patient's situation in his or her environment is an important component of many Step 3 questions. Laboratory values are given.

Clinical context of the Step 3 examination

The questions reflect clinical situations that a generalist physician might encounter, and they are written within the context of a specific setting. In addition, the items in each test book are arranged by the setting in which the encounter first occurs. On occasion, a patient encounter may begin in one setting and move to another. This is more likely to occur in case clusters.

When taking Step 3, you should assume the role of a generalist physician. Your office has regularly scheduled hours and includes a small laboratory for simple or routine tests. You admit patients to a 400-bed regional referral center. This hospital contains standard diagnostic, radiological and therapeutic options, including ICUs and cardiothoracic surgery. There is a labor and delivery suite. A fully equipped 24-hour emergency department adjoins the hospital. A medical evacuation helicopter service is available for emergency transfer to a larger tertiary-care teaching hospital. You do not have specialty-orientated hospital privileges, but you may request a specialty consultation.

Each test is divided into five sections that correspond to the clinical settings in which you will encounter patients. Each setting is described at the beginning of the section; they are outlined below.

Setting I: Satellite health center
This is a community-based health facility where patients seeking both routine and urgent care are encountered. Students from a nearby small university use the setting as a student health service. Several industrial parks and local small businesses send employees with on-the-job injuries and illnesses and for employee health screening. Usually the patients are being seen by you for the first time.

Setting II: Office
Your office is in a primary care generalist group practice located in a physician office near the local hospital. Most of the patients are your own scheduled, return visits, but occasionally you may encounter a patient whose primary care is managed by one of your associates. When a patient has a known history, it will be described as 'a history of drug abuse' or 'whom you have been treating for hypercholesterolemia'. Reference may also be made to the patient's medical records.

Setting III: Hospital
You have general admitting privileges to the hospital, including to the children's and women's services. On occasion you see patients in the critical care unit. Post-operative

patients are usually seen in their rooms unless the recovery room is specified. You may also be called to see patients in the psychiatric unit. There is a short-stay unit where you may see patients undergoing same-day operations or being held for observation.

Setting IV: Emergency department
Most patients in this setting are new to you. Occasionally, you arrange to meet there with a patient who has telephoned you. Generally, patients encountered here are seeking urgent care. Also available to you is a range of full social services, including rape crisis intervention, family support, and security assistance backed up by local police.

Setting V: Other encounters
You may be telephoned by a patient outside of office hours. Also, you may visit patients in their homes, nursing homes or extended-care facilities, such as the hospice, detoxification center or rehabilitation center. You spend time reading journals and interpreting the medical literature.

Item formats
Items are presented in three multiple-choice formats within each test book. Each of the formats requires selection of the one best choice. The general instructions for answering questions are as follows:

Single items
This is the traditional, most frequently used multiple-choice format. It usually consists of a description of a patient in a clinical setting, and a reason for the visit. The item vignette is followed by four or five response options lettered A, B, C, D and E. You are required to select the best answer to the question. Other options may be partially correct, but there is only ONE BEST answer.

Multiple-item sets
A single patient-centered vignette may be associated with up to three consecutive questions about the information presented. Each question is linked to the initial patient-centered vignette, but is testing a different point. Items are designed to be answered independently of each other. You are required to select the one best choice for each question.

The process for answering these items is the same as for single items. Items are usually phrased positively but occasionally they may be stated in the negative. Sometimes there will be one or more of each phrasing in a set. Pay particular attention when a negatively-phrased item is included.

Case clusters
A single-patient or family-centered vignette may ask as many as nine questions, each related to the initial opening vignette. Information is added as the case unfolds. It is extremely important to answer the questions in the order presented. Time often passes within a case and your orientation to an item early in a case may be altered by the additional information presented later in the case. If you do skip items, be sure to answer earlier questions with only the information presented to that point in the case. Each item is intended to be answered independently. You are required to select the one best choice to each question.

How to use this book
It is clearly not possible for a text of this kind (or any text for that matter) to cover all the material encountered in the actual examination. However, there are certain topics, mostly because of their special clinical importance, that are examined year after year. By working through this book we hope to familiarize you with the format of the examination and also to highlight areas that need further study in your overall preparation. In addition we have tried to cover favorite USMLE Step 3 topics.

There are two ways to work through this book. You can approach it piece by piece whenever you have the opportunity to study, focusing on 'weak' areas at a later time. Alternatively, and probably the better way, is to work through this book by simulating the examination. This latter way, by imposing a time constraint, helps to focus your study and to plan your time. As with all examinations, careful attention to time is of utmost importance.

Finally, we hope that this book will not only help with the examination, but will also help you in your practice of medicine. We welcome comments from readers.

Good luck!
Arshad Majid, MD

REFERENCE RANGES

Blood, plasma and serum

Parameter	Normal value
Amylase, serum	60–180 U/l
Bicarbonate, serum	21–30 mmol/l
Bilirubin, serum	0.1–1.0 mg/dl
Calcium, serum	9–10 mg/dl
Chloride, serum	98–106 mmol/l
CO_2 content, blood	24–30 mmol/l
Creatinine, serum	< 1.5 mg/dl
Dehydrogenase (lactate), serum	200–450 U/l
Electrolytes, serum	
Sodium	135–145 mmol/l
Chloride	98–106 mmol/l
Potassium	3.5–5.0 mmol/l
Bicarbonate	21–30 mmol/l
Folate, serum	6–15 ng/ml
Gases, arterial blood (room air)	
pO_2	75–100 mmHg
pCO_2	35–45 mmHg
pH	7.38–7.44
Glucose, plasma	
Fasting	70–110 mg/dl
2 h postprandial	< 140 mg/dl
Osmolarity, serum	275–295 mosmol/kg H_2O
Phosphatase (alkaline), serum	22–90 U/l
Proteins, serum	
Total	5.5–8.1 g/dl
Albumin	3.5–5.6 g/dl
Globulin	2.0–3.6 g/dl
Thyroxine (T_4), serum	4–12 µg/dl
Urea nitrogen, blood (BUN)	10–20 mg/dl
Uric acid, serum	3.0–7.0 mg/dl
Vitamin B_{12}, serum	200–600 pg/ml

Cerebrospinal fluid

Parameter	Normal value
Cell count	0–5 mononuclear cells/µl
Glucose	44–90 mg/dl
Pressure	10–20 cm H_2O
Total proteins	15–45 mg/dl

Hematologic

Parameter	Normal value
Hematocrit	
Male	42–52%
Female	38–46%
Hemoglobin	
Male	14–18 g/dl
Female	12–16 g/dl
Leukocytes	4500–10 000/µl
Neutrophils, band	1–20%
Neutrophils, segmented	26–63%
Lymphocytes	22–50%
Monocytes	2.4–11%
Eosinophils	0.3–5.0%
Basophils	0.6–1.5%
Mean corpuscular hemoglobin concentration	30–35 g/dl
Platelet count, blood	150 000–400 000/µl
Prothrombin time, plasma	< 2 s from control
Reticulocyte count	0.5–2.0%
Sedimentation rate, erythrocyte (Westergren)	
Male	0–15 mm/h
Female	0–20 mm/h

Urine

Parameter	Normal value
Creatinine clearance	80–140 ml/min
Osmolarity	48–1400 mosmol/kg H_2O
Protein	< 120 mg/24h
Specific gravity	1.002–1.028

TEST ONE

Satellite health center

1. A 50-year-old school teacher comes to your office for an annual check-up. He has no significant past medical history. He has been smoking a pack of cigarettes per day for 30 years and his father had been diagnosed with coronary artery disease when he was 50 years old. He is taking no medication other than multivitamins. Review of systems is otherwise negative. On physical examination his height is 5'10" and his weight is 184 lb. His pulse rate is 64 beats per minute and his blood pressure is 120/75 mmHg. His physical examination is otherwise unremarkable. You plan to order fasting lipids as part of your laboratory data. The goal for the LDL of this patient should be:

A. less than 200 mg/dl
B. less than 160 mg/dl
C. less than 130 mg/dl
D. less than 100 mg/dl

2. An 18-month-old is brought to your clinic by very distraught parents. The mother relates that shortly after checking the child's temperature (38.0°C), he had an approximately 5-minute event where he rhythmically moved all four extremities followed by a brief period of lethargy. After this they rushed the child to the clinic. The parents report no problems other than the fever and some irritability. Physical examination reveals a red, inflamed bulging right tympanic membrane, nontender neck with full range of motion and normal neurologic examination. You feel the child has a right otitis media and has experienced a febrile seizure. Your next course of action is:

A. obtain an EEG
B. admit the child to the hospital for evaluation and initiation of a prophylactic anticonvulsant
C. initiate prophylactic anticonvulsant therapy as an outpatient
D. obtain CT scan of brain
E. reassure and educate the parents that this is common and carries a good prognosis

3. During examination of any child, the medical caregiver should be vigilant concerning any of the features characteristic of the clinical picture for the child at risk for suicide. These risk factors include all of the following except:

A. increased prevalence of psychiatric disorders in parents and family
B. parental discipline of the child is inconsistent
C. child is socially isolated from peers and/or family
D. school performance is poor
E. child with chronic disease

4. A 5-year-old girl comes to your clinic with an acute onset of fever, emesis, pain on urination and abdominal pain. After physical examination your presumptive diagnosis is bacterial cystitis. Appropriate evaluation of this child's urinary tract infection includes each of the following except:

A. dimercaptosuccinic acid (DMSA) scan
B. renal ultrasound
C. intravenous pyelography
D. voiding cystourethrogram
E. percutaneous bladder tap for urine culture (suprapubic)

5. A 16-year-old girl is brought to your clinic by her parents. She has lost a large amount of weight in the past 8 months and has developed a moodier personality. Although she started her menses 2 years ago she has developed amenorrhea. Despite these changes her school performance has improved, she maintains a busy extracurricular schedule and a pristine appearance. When the girl is questioned she doesn't know what all of the fuss is about and states that her weight loss is secondary to a vigorous exercise program and new understanding of nutrition. Physical examination reveals a low normal heart rate, dry thin skin, dry hair with genital hair loss and decreased muscle mass. The most likely diagnosis is:

A. occult malignancy
B. inflammatory bowel disease
C. anorexia nervosa
D. hyperthyroidism
E. depression

6.   Breast-feeding offers a number of advantages to the newborn infant. There are few absolute contraindications to breast-feeding. One of them is:

A. galactosemia
B. maternal mastitis
C. Down syndrome
D. breast milk jaundice
E. pyruvate kinase deficiency

7.   A 16-year-old is brought in by her parents as they are concerned with her behavior after breaking up with a boyfriend 3 months ago. Her school performance has deteriorated, she complains of not sleeping well, she has lost weight and does not go out with her school friends as in the past. You ask the parents to leave so that you may talk with her alone. She denies any suicidal ideation, but does admit that she is having difficulty going to school and being motivated. She is not sure that she even wants her old boyfriend back at this time. Her physical examination is normal. Family history is not remarkable for suicide or psychiatric illness. The most appropriate action at this time is to:

A. reassure the parents that this is normal adolescent behavior and will resolve
B. have the parents remand the teenager to a military academy
C. admit the teenager for inpatient psychiatric therapy
D. refer the teenager and parents for counseling
E. initiate antidepressant therapy

8.   You receive a call from the state laboratory that performs the newborn screening tests. A child born 3 days ago has a positive test for phenylketonuria. You contact the family and arrange to see them immediately. Besides performing confirmatory laboratory studies you will:

A. tell the parents that their child will be severely mentally handicapped
B. initiate a low phenylalanine diet once the child has completed breast-feeding
C. refer them to a geneticist for counseling and therapy
D. initiate the child on a low phenylalanine diet immediately
E. refer them to a developmental specialist

9.   A 56-year-old black female presents with a history of a recent upper respiratory tract infection and red eyes, with the right eye involved first, followed by the left. The patient complains of a watery discharge, mild blurring of vision and no itching. On examination, small pinpoint subconjunctival hemorrhages and an enlarged preauricular node are noted. You would advise the patient all of the following except:

A. to observe good personal hygiene
B. the condition may worsen prior to improvement
C. to use artificial tears several times a day for 1–3 weeks, and cool compresses for symptomatic relief
D. this may be associated with pharyngoconjunctival fever
E. broad-spectrum topical antibiotics are the treatment of choice

10.   A 24-month-old child presents to your outpatient pediatric clinic with a white pupillary reflex noted on exam. Of the following etiologies that may contribute to such a presentation, the least likely would be:

A. retinoblastoma
B. retinopathy of prematurity
C. congenital cataract
D. histoplasmosis
E. toxocariasis

11.   A 28-year-old woman comes to your clinic requesting advice about prophylaxis against malaria. The following are useful in prophylaxis against malaria except:

A. use of bed-netting
B. wearing full-length clothes if possible
C. chemoprophylaxis according to the area of the world being visited
D. mosquito repellent
E. vaccination against malaria

12.   You are referring a 25-year-old woman for colonoscopy for altered bowel habit and bleeding per rectum. She reminds you that she has a heart murmur from mitral valve prolapse with regurgitation diagnosed by echocardiography. The most appropriate course of action is to:

A. tell the patient that the heart murmur is not important and the colonoscopy will not affect her heart
B. prescribe antibiotic prophylaxis against infective endocarditis before and after the procedure
C. tell the patient that the bowel problem and the heart problem are not linked
D. order a barium enema instead
E. order an echocardiogram before the colonoscopy

13–15. A 53-year-old woman comes to the office complaining of difficulty sleeping, generally feeling unwell and tells you that she may be going through the menopause.

13. Which of the following are laboratory features of the female menopause?

A. high follicle stimulating hormone (FSH) and low estrogen
B. low estrogen and low FSH
C. high estrogen and low FSH
D. high thyroid stimulating hormone (TSH)
E. high growth hormone (GH)

14. Which of the following is most commonly associated with menopause?

A. dyspareunia
B. major depression
C. panic attacks
D. brief psychotic disorder
E. generalized anxiety disorder

15. The woman in question is interested in HRT and wants to know more information about it. The following statements about HRT are correct except:

A. it provides protection against osteoporosis
B. it improves vaginal dryness
C. it decreases hot flashes
D. it decreases the risk of developing coronary artery disease
E. it increases the risk of developing uterine cancer

Office

16. A 2-year-old is brought to your office with pallor, lethargy, poor feeding and irritability. A microscope is available and his peripheral blood smear reveals a normocytic, normochromic anemia with no reticulocytosis. While awaiting the child's laboratory studies, your presumptive diagnosis is:

A. Diamond–Blackfan syndrome
B. autoimmune hemolytic anemia
C. glucose-6-phosphate dehydrogenase deficiency
D. aplastic anemia
E. transient erythroblastopenia of childhood (TEC)

17. A construction worker presents to your office complaining of decreased vision, photophobia, pain and discomfort after drilling wood at the job site. The patient denies any contact lens wear. Using fluorescein, you establish several vertical corneal abrasions in the left eye. At this juncture you should:

A. inform the patient of the etiology of his symptoms and place an antibiotic ointment and pressure patch and advise the patient to return in 24 hours
B. reassure the patient and apply a pressure patch and advise him to return in 24 hours
C. instill a cycloplegic to relieve the patient's symptoms and apply a pressure patch advising follow-up in 24 hours
D. advise the patient to wear protective eyewear and send him home with disposable sunglasses
E. evert the eyelids of both eyes, carefully inspecting for any foreign material that may be present with either irrigation or debridement followed by a complete dilated fundus exam

18. A 40-year-old white male presents to your office and complains of deterioration of his vision over the previous 3 days in the left eye. A relative afferent pupillary defect and blurring of the optic disc margin is established on examination. Of the following, the least likely association with this entity is:

A. decreased color vision
B. pain on eye movements
C. poor visual prognosis
D. potential risk for multiple sclerosis
E. history of a previous episode

19. A 4-month-old infant presents to your office for evaluation. The mother notes that her infant is not breast-feeding adequately despite repeated attempts. You notice epiphora (tearing) and redness in both eyes. You further ascertain that the infant exhibits blepharospasm. You should:

A. reassure the mother that this is an obstruction of the nasolacrimal duct and that it will resolve as the infant grows
B. inquire if the infant has exhibited this behavior over the past few months, particularly in well lit rooms
C. encourage the mother to supplement the breast milk with solid foods appropriate for age
D. consider working up the child for a metabolic disorder
E. refer the child to a pediatric neurologist to evaluate the blepharospasm

20. A 17-year-old is brought to your office by his parents, concerned that his school performance has deteriorated. Recently he has been diagnosed as intellectually limited. His parents insist that his grades had always been good until the last year. Over this year he has gained a significant amount of weight. When queried, his parents state that he snores so loudly that the whole house shakes. Physical examination is only remarkable for an obese, well-developed male with tonsillar hypertrophy. The likely diagnosis is:

A. obstructive sleep apnea
B. hypothyroidism
C. Cushing syndrome
D. mild mental retardation
E. learning disability

21. A 10-year-old boy is brought to your office. The parents explain that something is wrong with him. They relate that he can sit and watch his favorite television shows or play computer games for hours, but after 5 minutes in his school classroom he becomes disruptive. The mother shows you a note from the teacher stating that the child seems restless, cannot sit still, often does not complete assignments, and almost daily does something that disrupts the classroom. The physical examination is unremarkable, except that you note when you ask for his right arm or left arm the child seems confused before offering the appropriate extremity to you. The most appropriate diagnosis is:

A. Tourette syndrome
B. fragile X syndrome
C. conduct disorder
D. attention deficit hyperactivity disorder (ADHD)
E. cerebral palsy

22. Estrogen replacement therapy in postmenopausal women is associated with an increased risk of which of the following?

A. lung cancer
B. endometrial cancer
C. ovarian cancer
D. vaginal cancer
E. cervical cancer

23. A 67-year-old woman was treated by her primary care physician with courses of different antibiotics for a resistant chest infection. Two days after starting the third antibiotic she developed severe diarrhea. After appropriate testing, a diagnosis of *Clostridium difficile* enterocolitis (pseudo-membranous colitis) was made. *Clostridium difficile* entero-colitis can be treated with the following antibiotic:

A. metronidazole
B. erythromycin
C. gentamycin
D. cefotaxime
E. flucloxacillin

24. A 62-year-old African-American man presents to your office with his fourth attack of gout over the last month. The most appropriate initial treatment is:

A. intra-articular steroids and oral prednisone
B. oral aspirin 75 mg
C. furosemide
D. colchicine with allopurinol immediately
E. colchicine or indomethicin followed by allopurinol once the acute attack has settled

25. A 35-year-old Asian male presents with gross hema-turia and flank pain which has lasted for the last 24 hours. On further questioning he admits to having had some upper respiratory symptoms for the last 2–3 days. His past medical history is significant for an extensive workup for microscopic hematuria, which included a renal biopsy. Findings from biopsy samples included focal proliferative glomerulo-nephritis with predominantly mesangial cell proliferation by light microscopy, and globular deposits of immunoglobulins C3 and C5b9 in a predominantly mesangial distribution by immunofluorescence. His urinalysis was positive for protein and dysmorphic red blood cells and red blood cell casts, a 24-hour urinary protein collection showed a protein excretion of 2.7 g per day, his BUN was 25 mg/dl and his creatinine was 3.4 mg/dl. The most likely diagnosis is:

A. rapidly progressive glomerulonephritis
B. postinfectious glomerulonephritis
C. anti-glomerular basement membrane nephritis
D. IgA nephropathy
E. membranoproliferative glomerulonephritis

26. The following statements regarding venous thrombosis are correct except:

A. emboli are more likely to originate in calf veins than thigh veins
B. clinical diagnosis is often difficult and unreliable
C. venograms are helpful in the diagnosis
D. labeled fibrinogen scanning can help in the diagnosis
E. Doppler ultrasound is helpful in the diagnosis

27. A 27-year-old Indian woman had the following complete blood count:

Hb	13 g/dl
MCV	63 fl
MCH	25 pg/cell
MCHC	27 g/dl
WBC	$2.69 \times 10^9/l$
Platelets	$288 \times 10^9/l$
Hb electrophoresis	A, A2, F

The most likely cause of these hematological abnormalities is:

A. α-thalassemia
B. β-thalassemia trait
C. sickle cell anemia carrier
D. acute myeloid leukemia
E. chronic myeloid leukemia

28. Your advice to this patient if she were to have children with a β-thalassemia carrier would be:

A. there is a 25% chance that one of their offspring will have β-thalassemia major
B. all of their offspring will have β-thalassemia major
C. all of their offspring will be carriers of β-thalassemia
D. all of their offspring will have β- and α-thalassemia
E. there is a possibility that they will also have sickle cell anemia

29. A 26-year-old man is worried about an headache he had 2 hours ago at work. He describes a sudden-onset occipital headache, which lasted for 4–5 minutes and was the most severe headache he had ever had. There is no previous history of any other illnesses. Appropriate actions include:

A. referral to the emergency room for further investigation
B. prescribe painkillers in case he has a headache again
C. reassure the patient and tell him that it was probably a migraine and prescribe appropriate medications
D. ask him to call you immediately if the headache happens again
E. order an immediate erythrocyte sedimentation rate

30. He ignores your advice and attends the emergency room the next day. The initial emergency room investigations include all the following except:

A. CT and if this is negative, no further investigation
B. immediate MRI
C. CT and if this is negative, a lumbar puncture
D. immediate angiogram
E. PET scan

31–32. A 63-year-old ex-smoker of 2 years is concerned about the shape of his nails. Clinical examination shows marked finger clubbing.

31. This clinical sign is associated with the following disorders except:

A. bronchial neoplasm
B. chronic obstructive pulmonary disease (COPD)
C. bronchiectasis
D. cyanotic heart diseases
E. inflammatory bowel disease (IBD)

32. A few weeks later he was treated in hospital for pneumonia. At that time he also complained of excessive thirst, polyuria, weight loss, weakness and general malaise. On examination he was hypertensive (190/110), with a pulse rate of 90/min. The rest of the examination was normal.

Labs:

Na^+	146 mmol/l
K^+	2.3 mmol/l
BUN	10 mg/dl
Creatinine	1.0 mg/dl
HCO_3	38 mmol/l
Glucose	150 mg/dl

He was given dietary advice and discharged from hospital with a follow-up appointment to see an endocrinologist. Six months later he is admitted with increasing confusion, memory problems, agitation and difficulty with gait and coordination. Appropriate tests include all the following except:

A. anti-Hu antibodies
B. chest X-ray
C. MRI of the brain
D. CT of the chest
E. bone scan

33–39. A 68-year-old retired non-smoker comes to your office complaining of problems with his vision. On further questioning he describes a curtain coming down over his right eye for a period of 5–10 seconds and then disappearing.

33. After a full history and examination, appropriate first line investigation would include all the following except:

A. carotid duplex Doppler
B. EKG
C. EEG
D. complete blood count
E. carotid angiogram of the ipsilateral side to the symptoms

34. He undergoes a carotid duplex Doppler which shows greater than 90% stenosis of the right internal carotid arteries. This was confirmed by magnetic resonance angiography of the neck. The results of the North American Symptomatic Carotid Endarterectomy Trial (NASCET) showed that:

A. patients with 30–50% stenosis of the carotid artery benefited significantly from endarterectomy
B. only patients with greater than 90% stenosis benefit from endarterectomy
C. there is no conclusive evidence that endarterectomy is of any value
D. patients with symptomatic stenosis greater than 70% benefit from endarterectomy
E. all patients with greater than 70% stenosis should have endarterectomy

35. This patient was offered surgery but declined and decided on best medical management. All of the following have been shown to be useful in the prophylaxis against stroke except:

A. aspirin 75 mg
B. clopidogrel
C. ibuprofen
D. ticlopidine

36. The following are all associated with increased risk of stroke except:

A. hypertension
B. diabetes
C. dilated cardiac myopathy
D. atrial fibrillation
E. mitral valve prolapse

37. A few weeks later he presents to the ER with Broca's aphasia and right hemiparesis. Which vascular territory is likely to be involved?

A. right middle cerebral artery
B. basilar artery
C. posterior cerebral artery
D. anterior cerebral artery
E. left middle cerebral artery

38. Administration of tissue plasminogen activator (TPA) is considered. The National Institute of Neurological Diseases (NINDS) trial showed all the following about TPA except:

A. it increased cerebral hemorrhages 10-fold
B. it was ineffective if given within 2 hours
C. if administered within 3 hours, it increased by 30% the number of patients with little or no neurological deficit at 3 months
D. no overall increase in mortality in the treated group despite the increased number of hemorrhages

39. The following are all contraindications to tissue plasminogen activator (TPA) except:

A. witnessed seizure at stroke onset
B. only minor or rapidly improving clinical stroke
C. systolic BP > 185 and diastolic BP > 110 despite treatment
D. age over 75
E. lumbar puncture within 7 days

Emergency room

40. A 12-year-old boy is brought into the emergency department for recurrent seizures. There is no history of seizure disorder; however, there have been behavioral problems over the last 2 years, which include bed-wetting, and he had been prescribed a medication for this by a doctor while he was on holiday. Initial electrolytes showed a Na^+ level of 125 mmol/l and a K^+ level of 3.9 mmol/l. The rest of the laboratory investigations were normal. Possible drugs that may have caused this electrolyte imbalance in this boy include:

A. amitriptyline
B. furosemide
C. desmopressin
D. fluoxetine
E. chlorpromazine

41. Paramedics are bringing a 4-year-old who was playing in a field to the ER. His symptoms are described as muscle weakness, miosis, salivation and diarrhea, and now his heart rate is slowing down. Given his critical condition you want to be ready to start therapy immediately upon his arrival at the ER. Secondary to your presumptive diagnosis, upon his arrival you will initiate:

A. naloxone
B. atropine and pralidoxime
C. flumazenil
D. N-acetylcysteine
E. pyridoxine

42. A 2-month-old, known to have tetralogy of Fallot (TOF), is brought to the ER. Normally the child has an oxygen saturation of 90% on room air. The child is brought in by the parents owing to a hypercyanotic spell ('tet spell'). The child's current oxygen saturation is 55% (room air). The initial management steps for a hypercyanotic spell include the following except:

A. knee–chest positioning and 100% oxygen
B. 20 ml/kg of isotonic saline intravenous bolus
C. morphine sulfate (0.1 mg/kg intravenous bolus)
D. digoxin (5 μg/kg intravenous bolus)
E. phenylephrine (50–100 μg/kg intravenous bolus)

43. A 4-month-old is brought to the ER by his parents. They appear distraught. While watching their son sleep he had two periods of apnea requiring parental stimulation for resumption of breathing. The episodes were thought to last for a minute each and the child's color turned bluish. They woke the child and he has since been playful, interactive and appropriate for age. Past medical history is pertinent for the child being delivered at 34 weeks' gestation, although the child did well and was discharged at 5 days of life. Physical examination reveals a happy, interactive 4-month-old with no focal findings. Before stepping out of the room the parents relate that they are frightened. The appropriate next step is:

A. reassurance, education and discharge the family from the emergency room
B. after obtaining blood lab tests, reassure and educate the parents and send the family home
C. reassurance, education, and send the family home to follow up with their pediatrician
D. observe the child in the ER for 12 hours, then reassure, educate the parents and discharge home
E. admit the child to the hospital for observation, parental education and medical evaluation

44. A 38-year-old Asian female presents to the ER with marked pain, blurred vision and colored halos around lights with accompanying headache, nausea and vomiting. The patient relates a similar episode 1 month previously while at the movie theater that apparently resolved after going to the lobby. The findings associated with this entity include all of the following except:

A. may present as an acute abdomen
B. markedly elevated intraocular pressure
C. photophobia
D. corneal edema with conjunctival injection
E. normal pupillary exam

45. A 75-year-old black male presents to the ER with a complaint of painless visual loss in the right eye 2 hours earlier with an accompanying headache. You establish an afferent pupillary defect and with a clear view of the fundus on ophthalmoscopy, you notice a pale swollen disc with flame-shaped hemorrhages. The patient notes a significant decrease in vision (ability to count fingers) from a previous visual acuity of 20/20. On examination you notice tenderness over the right temporal artery. All of the following are appropriate, except:

A. obtain a neuroimaging study
B. inquire if there is any pain when chewing food
C. ask if there is any tenderness when combing hair, or with anorexia or fever
D. admit the patient and immediately initiate systemic steroids if you strongly suspect the diagnosis
E. obtain a stat erythrocyte sedimentation rate (ESR)

46. A 60-year-old patient is brought to the ER after sustaining a chemical burn to the right eye from an enraged spouse. You should immediately:

A. check the visual acuity
B. evert the eyelids and inspect for any foreign bodies
C. check the pH with a litmus paper, and then neutralize with either an acid or base solution as indicated
D. begin to irrigate copiously with saline solution
E. place a patch over the eye and contact an eye specialist for consultation

47. A 43-year-old patient found lying in a coma at home is brought to the ER. Serum potassium is 7.3 mmol/l but other electrolytes, as well as glucose, are normal. His EKG shows tall T waves but no other changes. Your most important immediate action is:

A. administration of intravenous calcium, intravenous insulin and dextrose
B. do nothing and repeat the electrolytes
C. get a renal ultrasound
D. start intravenous fluids and repeat electrolytes
E. get a renal consultation

48. A 55-year-old man enters the ER complaining of a 3-hour history of prolonged severe chest pain. He suddenly becomes unresponsive and the monitor shows ventricular fibrillation. After starting CPR, the most appropriate action would be:

A. defibrillate with 200 J
B. change the monitor and make sure the rhythm is correct before taking any further action
C. administer oxygen by face mask
D. administer atropine
E. administer norepinephrine

49. A 5-week-old male infant is brought to the emergency room with progressive non-bilious projectile vomiting over the past 48 hours. He is afebrile, and without diarrhea. Now he has decreased urine output and a dry mouth. The most likely diagnosis is:

A. viral gastroenteritis
B. gastroesophageal reflux
C. pyloric stenosis
D. appendicitis
E. constipation

50. A 47-year-old male presents to the emergency department with RLQ pain, which has progressed over the last 12 hours from a diffuse to a focalized discomfort. Recently, the patient has had complaints of episodes of flushing, occasionally combined with palpitations. Which of the following statements is true regarding carcinoid tumors of the appendix?

A. appendicitis is an uncommon presentation of appendiceal carcinoids
B. the size of the tumor is the best prognostic indicator
C. treatment for small (< 2.0 cm) carcinoids in the distal appendix is simple appendectomy
D. all of the above

51. Which of the following comments best describes the utility of a 24-hour urine collection for 5-hydroxyindoleacetic acid (5-HIAA) for the detection of carcinoid tumors?

A. highly specific, not very sensitive
B. not very specific, highly sensitive
C. not very specific or sensitive
D. only useful in detecting metastatic disease

52. A 65-year-old man with a 30-year history of symptomatic gastroesophageal reflux disease has had increasing dysphagia for solid food. An upper GI endoscopy reveals a 3.5 × 2 cm lesion of the distal esophagus, and biopsy specimens confirm the diagnosis of esophageal adenocarcinoma with surrounding areas of metaplasia consistent with Barrett's-type metaplasia. Which of the following statements is FALSE concerning esophageal adenocarcinoma?

A. medical treatment of gastroesophageal reflux disease decreases risk of esophageal adenocarcinoma
B. both duration and severity of symptoms are risk factors for the development of adenocarcinoma
C. some patients with invasive esophageal adenocarcinoma do not have Barrett's esophagus on biopsy
D. squamous cell carcinoma is more common than adenocarcinoma

Hospital

53. A 36-year-old woman undergoes sub-total thyroidectomy. Forty-eight hours after surgery, she starts complaining of muscle cramps and tingling in both her hands and feet. Appropriate treatment would include:

A. administration of thyroxine
B. administration of a β-blocker
C. administration of intravenous calcium
D. administration of intravenous glucose
E. administration of oral steroids

54. This woman returns for follow-up complaining of tiredness, feeling cold and generally unwell. She tells you that she has been taking her thyroxine following her surgery. Her blood tests show a grossly elevated thyroid stimulating hormone (TSH) but normal T_4.

A. the blood results indicate poor compliance with her medication
B. the results indicate hypothalamic failure
C. the results indicate that she needs more thyroxine
D. the results indicate that she has iodine deficiency

55. A 25-year-old patient presents to the ER with the rhythm shown (Figure 1). What is the rhythm shown?

A. atrial fibrillation
B. atrial flutter
C. atrial tachycardia
D. nodal rhythm
E. Wolff–Parkinson–White syndrome

56. This patient suddenly becomes unresponsive, with a BP of 50/30. The most appropriate action is:

A. synchronized DC shock at 50 J
B. intravenous amiodarone
C. unsynchronized DC shock at 100 J
D. synchronized DC shock at 200 J
E. intravenous thrombolysis as he may have had a pulmonary embolus

57. You are asked to see a 60-year-old patient whose main complaint is swelling and numbness of his upper and lower extremities. During your review of systems you find out that

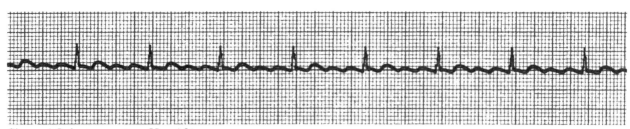

Figure 1 Refer to questions 55 and 56

he has been losing weight gradually over the past 2 years and that his exercise tolerance has markedly diminished over the last few months. Past medical history and family history are otherwise negative. On physical examination his heart rate is 80 beats per minute, and his blood pressure is 120/84 mmHg sitting and 100/80 when standing. His respiratory rate is 18. Examination of the head is significant for periorbital purpura, he has jugular venous distension, his chest is clear to auscultation, his heart sounds are regular and no additional murmurs are audible. He has hepatomegaly and a positive hepatojugular reflux; the rest of the abdominal examination is normal. His lower extremities have edema and there is a sensory deficit present. He has a positive Tinnel's sign. Echocardiography was interpreted as diastolic dysfunction due to left ventricular hypertrophy. All the following statements are true except:

A. most of his symptoms can be explained by diastolic dysfunction secondary to unrecognized hypertension
B. the most likely LFT abnormalities found in this patient will be a markedly raised alkaline phophatase with minimally elevated transaminases and bilirubin levels
C. ECG is likely to be read as prior silent myocardial infarction
D. urinalysis is likely to be positive for proteinuria

58. A 25-year-old obese woman seeks your advice about losing weight. Which of the following statements regarding obesity is false:

A. all adults with a body mass index of 25 or greater are considered at risk of developing associated morbidities or diseases such as hypertension, high blood cholesterol, diabetes mellitus and/or coronary artery disease
B. a body mass index of greater than 25 is indicative of obesity
C. presence of excess fat in the abdomen out of proportion to total body fat is an independent predictor of risk factors and morbidity
D. obesity-associated diseases include osteoarthritis, gallstones, stress incontinence and other gynecological abnormalities

59. Tricyclic antidepressants have the following properties except:

A. anticholinergic activity
B. cholinergic activity
C. they inhibit the uptake of norepinephrine
D. they are useful in the management of trigeminal neuralgia

60. You are called to perform a routine newborn examination on a 4-hour-old infant. There were no complications with the delivery. The physical examination is remarkable for a palpable 'clunk' of the right hip, upon abduction and internal rotation of the right leg at the hip joint. The appropriate management step is:

A. no therapy indicated
B. this is common; repeat examination at 1 week of age
C. instruct parents to place infant in double thickness diapers with the legs abducted and flexed
D. initiate use of a Pavlik harness
E. arrange for elective surgical correction

61. A 3-year-old is admitted with the presumptive diagnosis of meningococcemia. Earlier in the day the child was healthy and playful at his day care center. Now the child is intubated, on inotropic support, and receiving directed empiric antibiotic therapy. Shortly after arrival, the microbiology laboratory calls stating they see a large number of gram-negative diplococci on the Gram stain of cerebrospinal fluid. At this point you are confident the child has meningococcemia. What is the next step?

A. arrange for chemoprophylaxis of the family
B. notify the health department and arrange for chemoprophylaxis of family and day care center
C. notify the health department and arrange for immunoprophylaxis of family and day care center
D. arrange for chemoprophylaxis of health care providers and general hospital staff
E. no chemoprophylaxis is indicated

62. You are managing the care of a 73-year-old female patient in the surgical intensive care unit (SICU) who has been receiving TPN and is persistently ventilator-dependent. As part of a routine nutritional analysis, a respiratory quotient (RQ) was obtained, and the value is shown be 1.4. The most appropriate interpretation of this value in relation to her SICU care is:

A. the patient is protein malnourished, which can lead to decreased muscle strength
B. the patient is receiving inadequate carbohydrate and fat calories, which can cause increased CO_2 production
C. the patient is receiving too many calories, which can cause increased CO_2 production
D. the patient is receiving too many protein calories, which may be causing a metabolic acidosis

63. You are called to see a 54-year-old male who is postoperative day 1 from a splenectomy for ITP. There were no noted complications to the procedure. Just as you arrive in

the room the patient's blood pressure drops from 60/palpable HR 134 to no palpable pulse and an EKG which shows a narrow complex tachycardia. The patient is unresponsive and his extremities are cool to palpation. What is the most likely cause of his immediate state?

A. electrolyte abnormality
B. hypovolemia
C. myocardial infarction
D. embolism

64. A 65-year-old male with no significant previous medical history is seen by your office for jaundice and epigastric discomfort. A 4-cm hypoechoic mass is noted in the head of the pancreas on RUQ ultrasonography. The patient is otherwise healthy. Which of the following is the most appropriate next test in this patient's workup?

A. percutaneous biopsy under CT guidance
B. spiral CT
C. angiography
D. none of the above

65–68. A 34-year-old male is in the surgical intensive care unit (SICU) after a trip to the OR 3 days ago for multiple gunshot wounds to the abdomen, and an operative course that required resuscitation with 17 units of packed red blood cells, seven units of FFP, and two pooled units of platelets. Since returning from the OR he has demonstrated increasing difficulty with both ventilation and oxygenation. His chest X-ray (CXR) shows multifocal opacifications throughout all lung fields and he is ventilated with a pressure-control ventilation mode, receiving 80% oxygen. His ABG and PCWP this morning are:

pH	7.23
pO_2	56 mmHg
pCO_2	72 mmHg
HCO_3^-	12 mmol/l
PCWP	15 mmHg (NR 1–10)

65. Does this patient have adult respiratory distress syndrome (ARDS)?

A. no, his PCWP is too high to attribute his pulmonary failure to ARDS
B. no, his pO_2:FIO_2 ratio is too high to attribute his pulmonary failure to ARDS
C. no, his CXR is not consistent with ARDS
D. yes, he meets all the requirements for ARDS

66. You and your team are still evaluating the patient in the question above. Your chief resident says that he doesn't trust the recorded reading for the patient's PCWP and asks you to go into the room and reassess it. You enter the patient's room and carefully inflate the balloon catheter, look at the monitor and you notice that the PCWP varies between 14 and 18 with the patient's respiratory cycles. Which of the following statements is true regarding the accurate recording of PCWP in an intubated patient on positive-pressure ventilation?

A. the PCWP should be assessed at the lower number, when the patient is at end-expiration
B. the PCWP should be assessed at the higher number, when the patient is at end-expiration
C. the PCWP should be assessed at the lower number, when the patient is at end-inspiration
D. the PCWP should be assessed at the higher number, when the patient is at end-inspiration

67. Your patient from the previous question is now postoperative day 4, and his pulmonary status has acutely changed. This morning's chest X-ray shows improvement in his multifocal opacifications, but he is increasingly difficult to ventilate. He is on a pressure-controlled mode of ventilation, requiring peak inspiratory pressures in the range of 45–55 cm H_2O, to obtain a pCO_2 of 65 mmHg and a pO_2 of 76 mmHg on 60% FIO_2. His abdomen is tense and distended, and his urine output has dropped alarmingly from 50–75 cc/h yesterday to 5–10 cc/h today. His CVP is 13 cm and his PCWP is 20 mmHg. What would be an appropriate diagnostic maneuver to initiate at this point?

A. bronchoscopy
B. MRI
C. CT scan
D. measurement of bladder pressure

68. Your patient is likely to see some metabolic derangements as a result of the blood products that he received. Which of the following is NOT a common complication of massive transfusion?

A. increased left shift of oxygen/Hgb dissociation curve owing to increased pH
B. increased left shift of oxygen/Hgb dissociation curve owing to decreased 2,3-DPG in stored RBCs
C. impaired coagulation
D. hyperkalemia
E. all of the above are common complications of massive transfusion

69. A 33-year-old female is referred to your office for evaluation for possible familial adenomatous polyposis syndrome (FAP). Her father and grandfather both died of the disease, her father from a postoperative complication of a

total colectomy. On colonoscopy she was noted to have hundreds of small (< 0.5 cm) polyps, and several polyps in her sigmoid colon which are 1–1.5 cm. A protein truncation test (PTT) reveals that she carries a mutation in her *APC* gene that is known to be associated with FAP. Which of the following statements is FALSE regarding her condition?

A. colectomy should be performed only when a tissue diagnosis of adenocarcinoma is made
B. the average age of progression to symptomatic colorectal carcinoma (CRC) is 35 years of age
C. screening has been shown to decrease the average age of diagnosis
D. the disease is 100% penetrant

70–71. You are called upon to evaluate a 1-week-old infant in the nursery. There is evidence of a mucoid to muco-purulent discharge from both eyes with diffuse conjunctival injection and eyelid edema.

70. The following statements may pertain to this except:

A. gram-negative diplococci will be found in polymorpho-nuclear leukocytes on Gram stain
B. prescribe topical antibiotic ointment q.i.d., follow up daily until improvement noted
C. laboratory report indicates basophilic intracytoplasmic inclusion bodies in conjunctival epithelial cells
D. treat initially with erythromycin or ceftriaxone based upon the results of the Gram and Giemsa stains with modification according to the culture results
E. irrigate the discharge out of the fornices until removed, and obtain blood, viral and chocolate agar cultures from conjunctival scrapings

71. The etiology of this infant's presentation includes all of the following except:

A. *Chlamydia trachomatis*
B. *Neisseria gonorrhoeae*
C. *Escherichia coli*
D. staphylococci/streptococci
E. herpes simplex virus

72–73. You are called to see a 65-year-old male who was admitted for recurrent palpitations. On arrival at the bedside, the nurse tells you that the patient suddenly complained of shortness of breath and a BP measurement she has just done is 55/40. He is cold and clammy and poorly responsive. The EKG shows atrial fibrillation with a rate of 160 per second.

72. The most appropriate initial action is:

A. oral digoxin
B. saline
C. DC cardioversion
D. intravenous heparin only
E. intravenous heparin and intravenous digoxin

73. Recognized causes of atrial fibrillation include all of the following except:

A. thyrotoxicosis
B. mitral valve disease
C. coronary artery disease
D. embolic strokes
E. excessive alcohol consumption

74. You are covering the CCU and note the rhythm shown (Figure 2) on a monitor. The patient is short of breath and has some chest pain. His BP is 120/90. All the following drugs are helpful in managing this rhythm except:

A. lidocaine
B. atropine
C. amiodarone
D. procainamide

75. While you are deciding on the agent to administer this patient becomes unresponsive. The most appropriate immed-iate action is:

A. synchronized DC shock at 200 J
B. unsynchronized DC shock at 200 J
C. intravenous epinephrine
D. intravenous atropine
E. intravenous bretylium

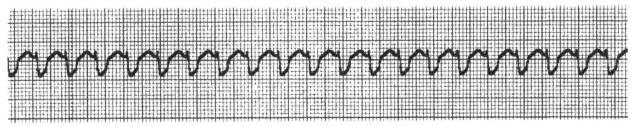

Figure 2 Refer to questions 74 and 75

Other encounters

76. Women with phenylketonuria (PKU) should be advised about the following:

A. low phenylalanine diet should be initiated as soon as pregnancy is confirmed
B. low phenylalanine diet should be started prior to conception
C. low phenylalanine diet is required in the third trimester
D. low phenylalanine diet has been shown to have no benefit during pregnancy
E. low phenylalanine diet should be followed in the first trimester

77. An 85-year-old woman presents to the office with a 2-day history of recurrent headaches and tenderness of the scalp. On further questioning she complains of a 6-month history of a general feeling of being 'unwell' associated with pain in her muscles. Appropriate first investigation would be:

A. CT of head
B. skull X-ray
C. erythrocyte sedimentation rate (ESR)
D. muscle biopsy
E. complete blood count

78. The following are all risk factors for endometrial cancer except:

A. obesity
B. diabetes
C. hypotension
D. late menopause and early menarche
E. ischemic heart disease

79. Which of the following workers are at the greatest risk of developing mesothelioma?

A. dentists
B. farmers working with pesticides
C. auto workers working on brakes
D. auto workers working with paints
E. miners

80. Maternal oligohydramnios is associated with:

A. umbilical hernia
B. esophageal or duodenal atresia
C. spina bifida
D. anencephaly
E. renal agenesis

81. Which of the following is the most common congenital heart lesion?

A. ventricular septal defect
B. patent ductus arteriosus
C. atrial septal defect
D. tetralogy of Fallot
E. transposition of the great arteries

82. The most common cause of a spontaneous pneumothorax is:

A. spontaneous rupture of a bleb
B. TB
C. bronchial neoplasm
D. trauma
E. asthma

83. The following are correct statements about breast milk compared to cow's milk except:

A. human breast milk contains more sodium, potassium and chloride
B. it contains IgA
C. it contains macrophages
D. it contains lysozymes
E. it contains lymphocytes

84. Which one of the following is NOT a characteristic feature of normal bereavement?

A. crying and tearfulness
B. decreased appetite with significant weight loss
C. social withdrawal and irritability
D. feelings of worthlessness and suicidal ideation
E. insomnia and decreased concentration

85. Which of the following is an example of highly adaptive defense mechanism?

A. rationalization
B. idealization
C. intellectualization
D. sublimation
E. withdrawal

86. During middle childhood, what behaviors are characteristic of each gender:

A. boys play in larger groups
B. boys in groups are more likely to interrupt one another, or call each other names
C. girls tend to form close friendships marked by the sharing of confidences
D. the breakup of a girl's friendship is more likely to result in intense emotional reactions
E. all of the above

87. All the following statements about guaiac-based fecal occult blood testing are true except:

A. stools containing hemoglobin levels of less than 1 mg/g can result in positive tests
B. fecal rehydration markedly raises the sensitivity of guaiac-based tests but reduces specificity
C. oral iron causes positive results on guaiac-based tests
D. diet modification is necessary when performing guaiac-based tests

88. Which of the following behavioral factors is NOT known to significantly increase the risk of developing esophageal adenocarcinoma?

A. smoking
B. alcohol use
C. nitrosamines
D. all of the above are risk factors
E. none of the above are risk factors

89. A 56-year-old man with a 3-year history of a venous leg ulcer complains that his wound has not been healing. You are interested in looking at factors that influence healing and tracking how well a wound is healing, and you find a study that compares the use of simple wound measurements (such as length or width) and computer-based planimetric measurement of the wound using a specialized tracing pen. This study provides both the parametric and non-parametric correlation coefficients between these two methods of wound measurement. A basic assumption behind all parametric methods is that:

A. the variable in question does not take on a negative value
B. the distribution is known
C. the standard deviation is less than 20% of the mean
D. all of the above
E. none of the above

90. The advantage of a parametric test over a non-parametric test is that it is:

A. easier to integrate with linear regression
B. more easily reproducible
C. more flexible for use with different types of data sets
D. none of the above
E. all of the above

91. You are interested in studying the risk of orthopedic injury in students playing competitive high-school sports. Reviewing the extant literature on this and related subjects, you find a recent article addressing the relative risk of head injury for students playing various high-school sports. The relative risk represents:

A. the incidence in the exposed group/the incidence in the unexposed group
B. prevalence in the exposed group/prevalence in the unexposed group
C. incidence in the exposed group – incidence in the unexposed group
D. prevalence in the exposed group – prevalence in the unexposed group
E. none of the above

92. After further consideration regarding your orthopedic injury study, you opt to conduct a case-control study design in order to save both time and money and in order to have a sufficient sample size. In this type of study, the relative risk (RR) may be calculated as:

A. approximated by the odds ratio
B. the incidence in the exposed group/the incidence in the unexposed group
C. the inverse of the odds ratio
D. prevalence in the exposed group/prevalence in the unexposed group

93. A 52-year-old man complains of lower back pain of 6 months' duration. You conduct a quick check of the literature and find a study on the treatment of lower back pain conducted at the New England Center for the Treatment of Lower Back Pain. The type of bias which would most concern you in this study would be:

A. recall bias
B. selection bias
C. interviewer bias
D. misclassification
E. none of the above

94. A 57-year-old woman complains of hot flashes. She states that she has seen several other physicians but that she is interested in alternative treatments for her condition. She then asks whether the fact that she has smoked one pack of cigarettes per day for the past 15 years would have any effect on her symptoms. She states that she heard about a study that enrolled 2500 women at the age of 35 and followed them until age 60 looking for the occurrence of hot flashes and other signs and symptoms of menopause (such a study does not exist). This type of study is best described as a:

A. prospective trial
B. clinical trial
C. cohort study
D. case-control study
E. none of the above

95. When discussing a similarly designed study with a colleague, she asks you why the investigators did not simply identify a group of patients with disease and then select a control group. The best response to this query would be that:

A. causality is better determined from cohort studies
B. cohort studies better demonstrate a temporal relationship between two events
C. cohort studies are cheaper
D. A and B
E. B and C

96. An 84-year-old man presents to your practice complaining of a 'funny-looking tongue'. On examination, you diagnose leukoplakia. You find an article discussing the association between leukoplakia and head and neck cancers, and in the course of reading you see that one of the associations has a *p* value of 0.052. The *p* value represents:

A. the probability that an effect at least as extreme as that observed could have occurred by chance
B. the probability that the association is due to chance
C. the probability that there is no relationship between the two factors
D. the probability that the results of the study are incorrect
E. none of the above

97. The *p* value in this study should be considered:

A. statistically significant
B. almost statistically significant
C. not statistically significant
D. clinically significant
E. none of the above

98–99. A patient approaches you and asks whether in your opinion drinking orange juice on a regular basis will help to prevent episodes of otitis media. As a mental exercise, you think about potential methods for designing a trial that would study this question. You decide that the best and least expensive way to conduct this trial would be to randomize patients and assign them to 4 weeks of drinking orange juice, and 4 weeks of drinking placebo, alternating back and forth for 24 weeks.

98. This study design is best described as a:

A. crossover study
B. clinical trial
C. case-control study
D. retrospective study
E. none of the above

99. This type of study assumes:

A. an effect is quickly obvious
B. there is no residual effect
C. a washout period would be included if there were concerns over a residual effect
D. all of the above
E. none of the above

TEST ONE: ANSWERS

1. Answer: C

The threshold serum total cholesterol and LDL cholesterol concentrations, above which diet and drug therapy should be initiated, as well as the goals of therapy, have been identified by the National Cholesterol Education Program. The target serum LDL cholesterol is less than 160 mg/dl for patients without risk factors, or with only one risk factor, for heart disease. The target is less than 130 mg/dl for patients with two or more risk factors, and less than 100 mg/dl for those with cardiovascular disease. Risk factors for cardiovascular disease identified by the National Cholesterol Education Program are: age (over 45 for men, after menopause for women), hypertension (even if treated), smoking, diabetes mellitus, history of cardiovascular disease in first-degree relatives (< 55 years of age for men, < 65 years of age for women), and serum HDL cholesterol of < 35mg/dl.

Reference: Knopp

2. Answer: E

Febrile seizures occur during both bacterial and viral infections. The children are typically between 6 months and 6 years of age. Simple febrile seizures last less than 15 minutes and are generalized. Complex febrile seizures last more than 15 minutes and may have focal ictal and post-ictal features. A good history and physical examination are important. Physicians must be able to comfortably rule out meningitis with their examination. Additional diagnostic studies are rarely indicated. The utility of an EEG, head CT or MRI, and lumbar puncture are very low. Occasionally, a serum glucose and chemistry are useful, but this is mostly in the situation where the underlying illness dictates that the child may have a metabolic disturbance. The question of long-term prophylaxis is a difficult one. One must consider the risk of recurrence of febrile seizures, versus the risk of the anticonvulsant medications. At this time most pediatric neurologists are not recommending or treating simple febrile seizures with anticonvulsants.

Reference: Oski et al., pp. 2058–61

3. Answer: D

Although poor school performance is a 'red flag', and may be an indicator of social or psychiatric difficulty, it is not one of the underlying characteristics in defining the clinical picture of a child at risk for suicide. Childhood suicide is described as self-inflicted death occurring before the fifteenth birthday. Important etiologies of suicide in adolescents are a major affective disorder, pre-existing chronic illness, drug abuse, schizophrenia and hysterical personality style or anti-social personality traits. The clinical picture that is characteristic of the child and family where suicide or attempts occur includes familial prevalence of psychiatric disorders, inconsistent discipline of the child, difficulty in emotional communication between family members, child with a psychiatric disorder, socially isolated child, and pregnancy or chronic illness of the child.

Reference: Oski et al., pp. 725–7

4. Answer: E

It is recommended that children with a documented urinary tract infection undergo evaluation of the anatomy of the urinary tract. A voiding cystourethrogram is used to evaluate the lower urinary tract. For evaluation of the upper urinary tract either a dimercaptosuccinic acid (DMSA) scan, intravenous pyelography, or renal ultrasound should be utilized. In a 5-year-old child the appropriate way to collect a clean urine culture is either via urethral catheterization or a midstream clean catch if the child and parents are co-ordinated enough. Generally, a percutaneous bladder tap is utilized in newborns and young toddlers as the bladder abdominal position is very anterior.

Reference: Zitelli and Davis, pp. 405–6; Oski et al., pp. 1770–2

5. Answer: C

Anorexia nervosa usually presents with clinical manifestations that when combined with an attentive patient and family history allow one to make the diagnosis. This includes her history and the clinical features of her examination. In addition, one can see bradycardia, hypotension, hypothermia, desquamating skin, and dry and thin vaginal mucosa. Additional features of the clinical picture include a family that displays little emotion and does not have good conflict resolution skills. Although the symptoms above can be consistent with inflammatory bowel disease, the lack of gastrointestinal complaints after an 8-month history is uncommon. It would be uncommon for a person with depression to have an improvement in school performance and a desire to maintain a pristine appearance with a busy extracurricular schedule. Hyperthyroidism is typically characterized by tachycardia, not a low normal heart rate.

Reference: Oski *et al.*, pp. 729–31, 797–802

6.   Answer: A

Infants with galactosemia cannot be breast-fed as galactose from any source is contraindicated. Current recommendations are to continue feeding through maternal mastitis and breast milk jaundice. Breast-feeding is not contraindicated in either Down syndrome or pyruvate kinase deficiency.

Reference: Zitelli and Davis, pp. 287–8; Oski *et al.*, pp. 596–601

7.   Answer: D

Physicians play a role in identifying adolescents and families that would benefit from counseling. Although she does not exhibit overt suicidal risks, she does have symptoms consistent with a dysfunctional parent/child relationship and persistent changes in behavior following stressful events. Since she does not have suicidal ideation at this time the best option is prompt referral for individual and family counseling. This may lead to pharmacologic management for depression if diagnosed.

Reference: Oski *et al.*, pp. 725–7, 738

8.   Answer: D

Phenylketonuria is an inborn error of metabolism where phenylalanine is not converted to tyrosine by phenylalanine hydroxylase. Early diagnosis via newborn screening has significantly altered the natural history of this disease. Once diagnosed, a diet that maintains the level of phenylalanine between 2 and 8 mg/dl must be initiated as soon as possible. Although dietary control does not restore neurologic dysfunction it will prevent further deterioration. At an appropriate time referral to a geneticist for counseling and possibly future prenatal diagnosis is indicated.

Reference: Oski *et al.*, pp. 85–7

9.   Answer: E

Viral conjunctivitis is contagious for up to 2 weeks. It can be preceded by an upper respiratory tract infection and also close contact with members of the family with a red eye. The involvement usually begins with one eye with subsequent involvement of the other eye shortly thereafter. Strict hygiene has to be observed to prevent spread. Supportive treatment is all that is needed for symptomatic relief of the patient's symptoms. Bacterial conjunctivitis is usually associated with mucopurulent discharge and unilateral involvement.

Reference: Wilson, p. 366; Vander and Gault, p. 48

10.   Answer: D

A white pupillary reflex is referred to as leukocoria. A number of entities must be kept in mind. Toxocariasis, a nematode infection involving the retina, usually occurs in children who have close contact with puppies or have a habit of eating dirt. Although the infection usually occurs between 3 and 10 years of age, it can also occur earlier in life. Retinoblastoma is the most common primary ocular tumor, in which 50% of cases present with leukocoria. Prompt recognition and treatment are essential given the risk for metastatic spread in the setting of orbital or optic nerve invasion. Congenital cataracts and retinopathy of prematurity also give rise to a white pupil. However, histoplasmosis is not a cause of leukocoria.

Reference: Vander and Gault, pp. 322–3; Cullom and Chang, pp. 181–3

11.   Answer: E

Malaria vaccination is not currently available although clinical trials are in progress. Decreasing skin exposure to mosquitoes by the use of bed netting and full-length clothing are useful measures. Mosquito repellents and chemoprophylaxis are also helpful.

Reference: Kelley, p. 1799; Rudy and Kurowski, pp. 758–9

12.   Answer: B

Prophylaxis against infective endocarditis is recommended for patients with aortic and mitral valve disease, VSD, coarctation of the aorta, patent ductus arteriosus, valves affected by previous endocarditis, hypertrophic cardiomyopathy and prosthetic valves. Prophylaxis against mitral valve prolapse is recommended if there is regurgitation. Patients with atrial secundum defects are thought to be at low risk and generally not thought to require prophylaxis.

Reference: Kelley, p. 1592

13.   Answer: A

High FSH and low estrogen are typical laboratory findings. There is no change in GH and TSH. Clinical features of the menopause include hot flashes, sweating, palpitations and dyspareunia due to vaginal dryness. Patients may also suffer from traumatic bleeding, stress incontinence and uterine prolapse.

Reference: Rudy and Kurowski, pp. 329–30

14.   Answer: A

Menopause was viewed in the past as a major etiological factor in mid-life psychiatric disorders in women. Research has established no firm links between menopause and any psychiatric syndrome, although there may be some evidence in favor of an association between hormonal replacement therapy and depression. Dyspareunia in females is commonly described as superficial pain during intromission or as deep pain during penile thrusting. The intensity of the symptoms may range from mild discomfort to sharp pain. This syndrome is frequently caused by the changes in secondary sexual characters associated with menopause (e.g. lack of vaginal lubrication or vaginal atrophy).

Reference: Hales and Yudofsky, p. 1270; DSM–IV, pp. 511–12

15. Answer: E

Unopposed estrogens can cause uterine hyperplasia and cancer. However, because most HRT treatments contain both estrogen and progestogen, the cancer-promoting effects of unopposed estrogens are not an issue.

Reference: Rudy and Kurowski, p. 334

16. Answer: E

TEC usually presents with pallor, poor feeding, lethargy, and irritability in children 1–4 years old. This is a transient and self-limited disorder characterized by a hemoglobin of 3–9 g/dl, normal mean corpuscular volume, inadequate reticulocyte count, normal white blood cell count and normal platelet count. TEC usually arises 2–4 weeks after a viral illness and may represent altered immunity from the infection that affects erythropoiesis. Both glucose-6-phosphate dehydrogenase deficiency and autoimmune hemolytic anemia would have evidence of hemolysis and a high reticulocytosis on peripheral blood smear. Diamond–Blackfan syndrome is chronic and usually presents in the first 6 months of life. Aplastic anemia involves other cell lines.

Reference: Zitelli and Davis, p. 314; Oski et al., p. 1668

17. Answer: E

Vertical abrasions should alert the physician that there may be foreign bodies underneath the tarsal conjunctiva of the upper or lower eyelid repeatedly rubbing against the cornea each time the patient blinks. It is imperative to evert the lids, inspect and irrigate the eye. A careful assessment of the fundus is also required to rule out vitreous hemorrhage or foreign body that may harbor microorganisms which may lead to endophthalmitis and loss of the eye.

Reference: Wilson, pp. 356–8

18. Answer: C

Optic neuritis, an inflammation of the optic nerve, typically occurs in the age range 18–45 years. It is usually unilateral and associated with pain on eye movement, acquired loss of color vision and an afferent pupillary defect. The loss of vision occurs over days with a visual field defect and a swollen disc on fundal examination. If vision is significantly decreased, the patient should be treated initially with intravenous steroids, not oral, as the latter increase the risk of recurrence. Though the etiology can be idiopathic, these patients are also at risk for multiple sclerosis later on in life. Over 90% of patients report pain with eye movement. The majority of patients will recover vision after noticing an initial decrement in visual acuity. Steroids hasten the rate of visual recovery. A similar presentation with a normal fundus exam should make one think of retrobulbar optic neuritis.

Reference: Berson, pp. 33–4; Vander and Gault, pp. 218–20; Cullom and Chang, pp. 274–6

19. Answer: B

Although nasolacrimal duct obstruction is common in infants, those presenting with a history of epiphora, photophobia, corneal edema and blepharospasm in association with a poor appetite, must be evaluated for congenital glaucoma.

Reference: Wright, p. 371; Cullom and Chang, pp. 202–4

20. Answer: A

Obstructive sleep apnea is characterized by enlarged tonsils and adenoids, upper airway abnormalities, hyperthyroidism and obesity. Associated symptoms include poor school performance, excessive daytime somnolence, nocturnal enuresis, morning headaches and changes in mood and personality. If not diagnosed and left untreated the patient may develop irreversible pulmonary hypertension and ultimately right heart failure. The differential diagnosis of any patient with marked weight gain in a relatively short period should include Cushing syndrome. The physical exam is usually remarkable for centripetal obesity, striae on skin, thinned skin, hypertension, weakness with muscle wasting, and moon facies. Elevated 24-hour urine free cortisol is the best diagnostic test. Hypothyroidism is characterized by obesity, constipation, cold intolerance, lethargy, delayed skeletal age and delayed puberty. Confirmatory tests include thyroid stimulating hormone (TSH), free T_4, T_4 and T_3 uptake.

Reference: Zitelli and Davis, pp. 270–2, 274–5; Oski et al., pp. 734–5, 1996–7, 2007–8

21. Answer: D

There is no specific test to diagnose ADHD and attention deficit disorder (ADD); only characteristic features obtained from a thorough history and physical examination allow you to make the diagnosis. Individuals with ADHD have difficulty sustaining attention and persisting to completion of a specific task. There is difficulty in organization and planning. In school this translates into a failure to complete assignments, difficulty waiting for their turn, inattentiveness during lectures, and interrupting others in the classroom. There may be subtle neurologic findings on examination, including difficulty of identification of right and left, difficulty with visual and sensory integration, dysdiadochokinesia, and synkinesis, with all of these persisting beyond the age of resolution (generally by 9 years of age). Diagnoses in the differential include static encephalopathy (cerebral palsy), mental retardation, early Tourette syndrome and personality/behavioral disorders.

Reference: Zitelli and Davis, pp. 71–2; Oski *et al.*, pp. 745–7

22. Answer: B

Administration of unopposed estrogens is associated with a significantly increased risk of endometrial cancer. The risk is related to the dose of administration and the duration. It is therefore recommended that women who have not undergone hysterectomy take progestogens with estrogen.

Reference: Rudy and Kurowski, p. 337

23. Answer: A

Virtually all antibiotics can cause pseudomembranous colitis, but particular offenders are penicillins, cephalosporins and clindamycin. Appropriate action in this case would be cessation of the offending antibiotic and treatment with the appropriate agent. Oral vancomycin, metronidazole and bactricin are effective treatments against *Clostridium difficile*. Vancomycin should be reserved for resistant cases. In mild cases antibiotic treatment may not be necessary.

Reference: Kelley, pp. 1676–7

24. Answer: E

The most appropriate line of treatment for this patient is either colchicine or indomethicin for the acute episode. Once the inflammation has resolved, an agent that will lower his uric acid levels such as allopurinol should be used as prophylaxis. Use of allopurinol during an acute attack of gout can precipitate or prolong the acute episode. Intra-articular glucocorticoids and oral prednisone can be useful when colchicine and NSAIDS are contraindicated.

Reference: Rudy and Kurowski, p. 423

25. Answer: D

In developed countries, IgA nephropathy has replaced poststreptococcal glomerulonephritis as the leading cause of glomerulonephritis, and because of its high prevalence in Asian countries, it is probably the most common cause of glomerulonephritis worldwide. Fifty per cent of patients present with primary renal disease, commomly as abrupt onset of gross hematuria, 24–48 hours after an upper respiratory or gastrointestinal infection. Protein excretion is increased but rarely exceeds 3.5 g per day, and renal function

is commonly impaired during acute episodes that last 6–8 days. Edema and hypotension are much less common than in poststreptococcal glomerulonephritis. Approximately 30–40% develop persistent microscopic hematuria. Renal biopsy findings are consistent with proliferative glomerulonephritis, with predominantly mesangial cell proliferation by light microscopy. Globular deposits of IgA, C3 and C5b9 in a predominantly mesangial distribution are found on immunofluorescence.

Reference: Durand

26. Answer: A

Doppler ultrasound and venograms are helpful in the diagnosis of deep venous thrombosis. Radioactive fibrinogen scanning can also help in the diagnosis but is not routinely used in clinical practice. Clinical diagnosis is difficult and often only detects 50% of confirmed deep venous thrombosis. Emboli are more likely to originate from the thigh veins than the calf veins. The incidence of pulmonary emboli is underestimated.

Reference: Rudy and Kurowski, pp. 109–16

27. Answer: B

Beta-thalassemia trait (minor). The severe microcytosis in the absence of anemia in this patient of Indian origin suggests either β- or α-thalassemia traits are possible diagnoses. However, to help us further, elevated Hb A2 and Hb F are given which indicates that β-thalassemia trait is the likely diagnosis.

Reference: Kelley, pp. 1440–1

28. Answer: A

Beta-thalassemia is inherited in an autosomal recessive manner. Therefore there is a 25% chance that one of their offspring will have β-thalassemia major.

Reference: Kelley, pp. 2283–302

29. Answer: A

Sudden-onset severe headache is a classical history for subarachnoid hemorrhage (SAH) and this diagnosis needs to be ruled out immediately. Having one SAH puts the patient at increased risk of another SAH.

Reference: Rudy and Kurowski, pp. 124–5

30. Answer: C

A CT will pick up greater than 90% of subarachnoid hemorrhages (SAH) and a CT with an LP will pick up over 95% of SAH. An MRI is an insensitive test for acute bleeds. PET scanning has no role in acute management of SAH. If SAH is confirmed, then MR angiography or conventional angiography would be the next investigation to look for aneurysm and arteriovenous malformations.

Reference: Rudy and Kurowski, pp. 124–5

31. Answer: B

Clubbing, which constitutes increased curvature of the nail, loss of nail bed angle, and fluctuation of the nail bed on palpation, is not associated with COPD. Other associated conditions include pulmonary fibrosis and infective endocarditis.

Reference: Bates, p. 145

32. Answer: E

The history and presentation suggest a paraneoplastic syndrome. The confusion, memory problems and agitation suggest limbic encephalopathy. Other features include cerebellar and brain stem dysfunction and sensory neuropathy. Anti-Hu antibody titers may be raised in these patients and are helpful in the diagnosis, especially if a primary lesion is not found. The most common tumor associated with this condition is small cell carcinoma of the lung. Other tumors include prostate cancer, neuroblastoma and chondromyxosarcoma. Paraneoplastic antibody syndromes may pre-date the 'appearance' of the tumor by months or years. There is no effective treatment, although treatment of the primary lesion may stabilize the neurological symptoms.

Reference: Kelley, pp. 2051–2

33. Answer: C

This patient is describing amaurosis fugax, a type of transient ischemic attack. Appropriate investigations initially would include carotid duplex Doppler, EKG, complete blood count, electrolyte lipid profile and CT. This history is not suggestive of seizures, so an EEG is not indicated.

Reference: Samuels and Feske, p. 43

34. Answer: D

The NASCET showed that symptomatic patients, i.e. those with a previous stroke or TIA ipsilateral to 70% or greater stenosis, benefited from endarterectomy following a 2-year follow-up period. There is also evidence from the Asymptomatic Carotid Artery Stenosis Study (ACAS) that asymptomatic patients with greater than 60% stenosis benefit from carotid endarterectomy. However, the relative benefit of endarterectomy is much greater in the symptomatic patients with greater than 70% stenosis.

Reference: Samuels and Feske, pp. 344–5

35. Answer: C

A number of studies have shown the benefit of aspirin in the secondary prevention of stroke. More recently, ticlopidine, dipyridamole and clopidogrel have also been shown to be efficacious. Ibuprofen has not been shown to be of value in the prevention of stroke.

Reference: Samuels and Feske, pp. 342–44

36. Answer: E

Hypertension and diabetes are well recognized modifiable risk factors for stroke. Atrial fibrillation and dilated cardiomyopathy increase the risk of embolic stroke. No clear association between mitral valve prolapse and stroke has been found unless there is myxomatous change of the valve.

Reference: Samuels and Feske, p. 331; Kelley, p. 446

37. Answer: E

In over 90% of right-handed and over 60% of left-handed people, the left hemisphere is language dominant. The right hemiparesis and Broca's aphasia suggests a cortical stroke affecting the left middle cerebral artery territory.

Reference: Samuels and Feske, p. 337

38. Answer: B

The NINDS study showed that despite the 10-fold increase in intracranial hemorrhages, patients treated with intravenous TPA within 3 hours of onset of symptoms were 30% more likely to have little or no deficit at 3 months. In addition, there was no difference in overall mortality between the two groups despite the increased number of hemorrhages in the treated group.

Reference: Cummins, p. 10.15

39. Answer: D

TPA is not licensed for patients under 18 but there is no upper age limit. Witnessed seizure, uncontrolled hypertension, minor stroke, LP in the last 7 days, and major trauma or surgery in the last 14 days are all contraindications. Other contraindications include, but are not limited to, bleeding diathesis.

Reference: Cummins, p. 10.16

40. Answer: C

Desmopressin has been found to be useful in nocturnal bed-wetting in children but hyponatremia is a recognized side-effect. Seizures caused by hyponatremia is the likely answer. Amitriptyline overdose can also cause seizures but not the reported electrolyte abnormalities.

Reference: Fauci et al., p. 169

41. Answer: B

Organophosphate poisoning is the leading cause of nonpharmaceutical ingestion fatality in children. Organophosphates are absorbed across skin and mucous membranes, binding irreversibly to neuronal and erythrocyte cholinesterase and to liver pseudocholinesterase. This results in a failure to terminate the effects of acetylcholine at central cortical, respiratory and cardiac centers, and peripherally at nicotinic and muscarinic receptors. The therapies of choice are atropine and pralidoxime. Naloxone is the reversal agent for opioid overdose. Flumazenil is the antagonist for benzo-diazepines. N-acetylcysteine is the treatment of choice for acetaminophen overdose. Pyridoxine is the therapy for isoniazid.

Reference: Oski *et al.*, p. 836

42. Answer: D

TOF refers to a congenital heart lesion characterized by ventricular septal defect, right ventricular outflow tract obstruction, overriding aorta and hypertrophy of the right ventricle. TOF is found in approximately 6% of infants born with congenital heart disease. Episodes of paroxysmal hypoxemia, known as hypercyanotic episodes or tetralogy spells, are often seen in infants with TOF. The physiologic change that occurs is increased right-to-left shunting, resulting in a decrease in pulmonary blood flow. These spells usually last 15–30 minutes, but they can last longer and can result in death. These spells should be treated aggressively, and if not readily responsive to therapy are an absolute indication for corrective surgery. Interventions that are appropriate include knee–chest positioning of the child (increases systemic vascular resistance resulting in greater pulmonary blood flow), 100% oxygen, isotonic volume expansion, morphine sulfate, phenylephrine and propranolol.

Reference: Oski *et al.*, pp. 1536–8

43. Answer: E

An infant who experiences a severe ALTE should be monitored in the hospital for 48 hours (minimum) after the event. Hospitalization allows for close observation, cardio-respiratory monitoring, parental education, and appropriate medical studies if indicated. Many parents are very frightened by these events and therefore the child may require a short hospitalization for reassurance and education. Conditions associated with ALTEs include cardiac disease, respiratory disease, gastroesophageal reflux, anemia, hyper-ventilation, neurologic disorders, metabolic disorders and prematurity.

Reference: Oski *et al.*, pp. 1058–64

44. Answer: E

Angle closure glaucoma is common in Asians and Eskimos. The fact that this patient had a similar episode in the dark indicates that when the pupil dilates to allow more light into the eye, the iris narrows the angle further, creating an attack. By constricting in the lighted area (the lobby), the narrowing phenomenon is reversed. Such an acute attack can mimic an acute abdomen with nausea and vomiting. The pupil is typically dilated due to the markedly elevated eye pressure with ischemia to the sphincter muscle that constricts the pupil.

Reference: Vander and Gault, pp. 121–2; Cullom and Chang, pp. 226–9

45. Answer: A

Giant cell arteritis is an emergency and predominantly occurs after the sixth decade of life. There is associated visual loss and a 30–40% risk of involving the contralateral eye if intervention with high-dose systemic steroids is not immed-iately instituted. It can be associated with jaw claudication, scalp tenderness, proximal muscle weakness, anorexia, weight loss or fever. The ESR is usually but not always markedly elevated. Examination findings include a palpable tender temporal artery. Temporal artery biopsy showing arteritis is the gold standard test. Neuroimaging is not indicated.

Reference: Vander and Gault, pp. 222–3; Berson, pp. 35–6

46. Answer: D

First and foremost, the eye has to be irrigated copiously, especially given that alkaline solutions continue to damage the ocular tissue and penetrate into the deeper layers with risk for intraocular complications. Acid burns cause protein denaturation that subsequently acts as a barrier to the diffusion of the chemical and thus limits the degree of damage. One should also thoroughly irrigate the fornices. Recommended time of irrigation is up to 30 minutes either manually or with IV tubing connected to an irrigation appa-ratus. Only after waiting at least 5 minutes after irrigation is completed to allow for equilibration should the pH be assessed by litmus paper. Irrigation should be continued until neutralization is established.

Reference: Vander and Gault, p. 54; Wilson, pp. 369–70

47. Answer: A

The potassium level of 7.3 mmol/l is a medical emergency and requires immediate action. This involves administration of intravenous calcium, which antagonizes the effect of potassium on the myocardium. Insulin and glucose will shift potassium to the extracellular space. Exchange resins will reduce total body potassium but take time to take effect. Other treatments include diuretics and dialysis. The EKG changes of tall T waves are consistent with hyperkalemia.

Reference: Kelley, p. 966

48. Answer: A

The history suggests that the patient is having or has had a myocardial infarct. Ventricular fibrillation is the most freq-uent initial rhythm after sudden cardiac arrest. The only effective treatment for ventricular fibrillation is defibrillation and the probability of successful defibrillation diminishes over time. The most appropriate immediate action would be defibrillation with 200 J.

Reference: Cummins, p. 4.1

49. Answer: C

The classic presentation of pyloric stenosis is a 3–6-week-old male infant with progressive non-bilious projectile vomiting leading to dehydration with hypochloremic, hypokalemic, metabolic alkalosis. On physical exam a pyloric 'olive' is palpable and peristaltic waves are visible. If the diagnosis is in doubt, ultrasound can be used to visualize the hypertrophic pyloric musculature. Appendicitis does not usually present at this age, and a fever is usually present. Gastroenteritis usually has diarrhea associated with emesis. Constipation does not generally result in vomiting. Gastroesophageal reflux is self-limited and does not result in dehydration.

Reference: Zitelli and Davis, pp. 293–5; Oski *et al.*, p. 418

50. Answer: D

Carcinoid tumors are the most common primary tumors of the appendix, occurring most commonly in patients 40–60 years old. Appendicitis is an uncommon presentation for a carcinoid tumor – these tumors occur 75% of the time in the distal appendix (only 10% of the time at the base), and are therefore usually unable to obstruct the appendiceal lumen and cause appendicitis. The size of these tumors is the best prognostic factor – there are only rare instances of tumors < 2.0 cm as a source of metastatic disease. The treatment for tumors < 2.0 cm in the distal appendix is simple appendectomy. Larger tumors are best treated with right hemicolectomy.

Reference: Kulke and Mayer

51. Answer: D

The urinary screen for serotonin metabolites is a highly sensitive (73%) and specific (100%) test for the detection of metastatic carcinoid disease. However, most patients with carcinoid tumors and no carcinoid syndrome will have normal levels of 5-HIAA, limiting its value as a screening tool.

Reference: Kulke and Mayer

52. Answer: A

Both duration and severity of symptoms are independent risk factors for the development of esophageal adenocarcinoma. Patients with severe reflux symptoms have a risk level for the development of adenocarcinoma that is 20 times greater than patients without reflux symptoms. Only 62% of patients with esophageal adenocarcinoma have Barrett's. Squamous cell carcinoma accounts for approximately 90% of esophageal carcinomas, with esophageal adenocarcinoma making up the bulk of the remaining tumors. There is no indication that medical therapy (H_2 blockers, proton pump inhibitors) decreases risk for development of esophageal adenocarcinoma.

Reference: Lagergren *et al.*

53. Answer: C

Her symptoms are due to hypocalcemia caused by hypoparathyroidism. The parathyroids were removed during her surgery and appropriate initial treatment would be intravenous calcium. Oral calcium and vitamin D should be administered long-term.

Reference: Fauci *et al.*, p. 2166

54. Answer: A

The elevated TSH and normal T_4 indicate poor compliance with her medication. The normal T_4 indicates that she has recently taken thyroxine, possibly on the day of the blood test. The elevated TSH excludes hypothalamic failure. These results give no indication of iodine deficiency. She may need more thyroxine replacement but this needs to be assessed when compliance to treatment is established.

Reference: Kelley, p. 2214

55. Answer: B

The rhythm strip shows atrial flutter with the characteristic 'saw-tooth' baseline with a normal-looking QRS complex.

Reference: Cummins, pp. 3.11, 4.6

56. Answer: A

The immediate treatment in this patient is synchronized DC shock at 50 J. If this is unsuccessful 100 J and then stepwise increments are recommended. In atrial fibrillation 100 J should be the starting energy.

Reference: Cummins, pp. 3.11, 4.6

57. Answer: A

This patient has amyloidosis. This diagnosis should be considered in older patients who present with nephrotic syndrome, hepatomegaly, congestive heart failure and/or peripheral neuropathy. If diabetes and hypertension are excluded, amyloidosis is found in 10% of patients with adult onset nephrotic syndrome. Hepatomegaly is commonly due to congestive heart failure; 25% of patients will have infiltration of their liver characterized by markedly increased alkaline phosphatase and by minimally increased bilirubin and transaminases. Cardiac involvement is characterized by congestive heart failure. The diagnosis should be suspected in any patient with no history of ischemia or major risk factors for coronary disease. The ECG can be misleading owing to a pseudoinfarction pattern. Echocardiography represents the standard test for all patients in assessing the presence or absence of amyloid; however, it is commonly misinterpreted as left ventricular hypertrophy. Overt congestive heart failure is the most powerful prognostic factor. Neurological manifestations of amyloidosis are: peripheral neuropathy, concomitant presence of a carpal tunnel syndrome as well as autonomic neuropathy manifested by diarrhea, orthostatic hypotension, or unexplained nausea or vomiting.

Reference: Gertz *et al.*

58. Answer: B

The body mass index, which describes relative weight for height, is calculated as weight in kilograms divided by height in meters squared. Classification of overweight and obesity by body mass index is the following: a body mass index of less than 18.5 is considered underweight, 18.5–24.9 is normal, 25.0–29.9 is overweight and greater than 30 is obese.

Reference: Executive summary

59. Answer: B

Tricyclic antidepressants have anticholinergic activity and have common side-effects related to this. Their main mechanism of action is inhibition of norepinephrine uptake. They have been also found to be useful in the treatment of neuropathic pain such as trigeminal neuralgia.

Reference: Rudy and Kurowski, p. 800

60. Answer: D

Congenital dislocation of the hip is a relatively frequent problem, occurring in 1–2 per 1000 births. The initial physical examination of a newborn infant should include two maneuvers: Ortolani's and Barlow's tests. Ortolani's test is positive when a palpable clunk is felt upon abduction and internal rotation of the hips. Barlow's test is positive if, with the knees and hips flexed at 90°, the hips are adducted with pressure applied on the lesser trochanter. A palpable clunk occurs with posterior dislocation of the hip. Both radiographs and ultrasound of the hips can be useful in confirming the clinical diagnosis. Dislocated hips should be treated at the time of diagnosis. A hip abduction and flexion device such as a Pavlik harness should be used. After one week of therapy alignment should be checked via radiography. Generally therapy will last 2–4 months. Occasionally a child may still require surgical correction after wearing the harness.

Reference: Zitelli and Davis, pp. 665–7; Oski *et al.*, pp. 1018–20

61. Answer: B

Meningococcemia is caused by *Neisseria meningitidis*, a gram-negative coffee bean-shaped diplococcus. Meningococcemia constitutes a medical emergency. Aqueous penicillin G remains the drug of choice. Chemoprophylaxis is recommended for household members and day care center contacts that are toddlers or younger (secretion-sharing age groups). It is also recommended that the index patient receive treatment to eradicate the carrier state. Immunoprophylaxis is recommended for people with anatomical or functional asplenia and deficiencies of the complement system. In addition, travelers to hyperendemic or epidemic areas should receive the immunization.

Reference: Oski *et al.*, pp. 1199–203

62. Answer: C

The RQ is determined by assessing CO_2 produced and O_2 consumed. Metabolic reactions that generate a high amount of CO_2 relative to O_2 consumed have a high RQ, and the converse reactions have a low RQ. The conversion of glucose to fat generates CO_2 in the absence of a significant O_2 consumption. This patient's high RQ is indicative of a state of overfeeding.

Metabolic pathway	*RQ*
Carbohydrate metabolism	1.0
Fat metabolism	0.7
Protein metabolism	0.8
Glucose conversion to fat	8.0

Reference: Greenfield, pp. 1044–5

63. Answer: B

Electromechanical dissociation (also known as EMD, pulseless electrical activity (PEA), pseudo-EMD) may be caused by a wide variety of factors, including hypovolemia, hypoxia, MI, tamponade, pulmonary embolism and many more. The most common cause of EMD is hypovolemia. This cause is especially likely in a patient that is post-splenectomy, as this procedure involves the manipulation and ligation of the short gastric arteries between the stomach and the spleen; intra-abdominal bleeds are a common post-operative complication.

Reference: Cummins, p 1.21

64. Answer: B

The next step in this patient's workup is to determine resectability of the presumed malignancy. Percutaneous biopsy is considered an unnecessary test in this patient's workup as he is a good operative risk. A patient that is a poor risk, with an unresectable mass, may benefit from a tissue diagnosis in order to direct chemoradiation therapy. Spiral CT, MRI, and endoscopic ultrasound (EUS) are considered the best tests to stage pancreatic tumors and determine resectability. EUS is considered a superior test for smaller tumors (< 3 cm) but spiral CT is a better test for larger tumors and for assessing nodal and other metastases. Angiography frequently overestimates the extent of vascular invasion because local tissue response to tumors can simulate vascular invasion.

Reference: Yeo and Cameron

65. Answer: B

The European Consensus group has dictated three major requirements for a patient to be classified as having ARDS: 1) pO_2:FIO_2 < 200; 2) PCWP < 18; and 3) CXR consistent with ARDS. This patient's CXR and PCWP are consistent with ARDS, but his oxygenation is still too good to give him the classification of ARDS.

Reference: Bernard *et al.*

66. Answer: A

A complete discussion on accurate interpretation of invasive hemodynamic monitoring is beyond the scope of this question's explanation. However, this question illustrates an important point: the distinction between intravascular and transmural pressures. Imagine diving to 100 m below the sea – the effect would be an effective increase in measured intravascular pressure, but not transmural pressure. A state of pulmonary edema from elevated central venous pressures would not occur. The same phenomenon occurs with positive pressure ventilation – throughout the respiratory cycle the ventilator induces a high pressure state in the thoracic cage. This externally applied pressure is lowest at end-expiration, and it is at this point that the PCWP should be assessed. Note that if positive end-expiratory pressure (PEEP) is being applied, then this pressure will also influence PCWP. The most accurate assessment of PCWP would occur with PEEP temporarily turned off.

Reference: Marino, pp. 166–8

67. Answer: D

Abdominal compartment syndrome (ACS) is a common sequela of the type of injuries and management in this situation. Abdominal surgery with primary closure in the face of massive intra-abdominal injury frequently leads to increased intra-abdominal pressure, which will eventually lead to ACS. The syndrome manifests itself as a tense abdomen, decreased renal function and venous return, and difficulty with ventilation and oxygenation as a result of increased abdominal pressures transmitted to the thorax. Bladder pressure has been shown to be an accurate surrogate of intra-abdominal pressure, and pressures greater than 20 cm H_2O are strongly associated with ACS.

Reference: Ivatury *et al.*

68. Answer: E

Blood transfusions are by no means a risk-free undertaking. Their adverse effects are manifold, and are implicated in adult respiratory distress syndrome and impaired immunologic function. Many of the more severe metabolic effects are not seen until massive levels of transfusion occur, as in this patient. Citrate is used as one of the preserving agents, to bind calcium thereby inhibiting the coagulation cascade at several points. The infusion of the large citrate load can bind calcium out of the intravascular space, causing hypocalcemia and coagulopathy. Even though stored blood has an acid pH, the citrate preservative is converted to bicarbonate

in the liver, and this can contribute to an increased pH. In blood products that are near the end of their storage life, concentrations of 2,3-DPG are lower owing to cellular metabolism, and large-scale infusion of these RBCs (functioning with a left-shifted oxygen/hemoglobin dissociation curve) can lead to decreased delivery of oxygen to tissues. The concentration of potassium in stored blood rises during its storage, and can be as high as 40 mmol/l, a potential cause of hyperkalemia.

Reference: Sabiston, pp. 118–25

69. Answer: A

Five per cent of patients with FAP develop CRC by age 20. The genetic test (protein truncation test) for *APC* mutations is able to pick up 80% of mutations, and it is therefore a reasonable test to establish the diagnosis of FAP. The average age of presentation with symptoms that prove to be related to FAP is 35 years of age; patients with a strong family history of FAP that undergo intensive screening are identified significantly earlier. The disease shows an autosomal dominant pattern of inheritance, and a 100% penetrance. Prophylactic colectomy is therefore more strongly indicated for FAP.

Reference: Guillem *et al.*

70. Answer: B

The presence of ophthalmia neonatorum (newborn conjunctivitis) requires prompt and appropriate therapy. Otherwise, there is a risk not only for penetration of the cornea and ocular involvement but for compromise of the infant as well, with systemic involvement. It is not sufficient to treat the eye infection with topical antibiotics, for there is a potential for disseminated disease. Infants are at risk for developing otitis media and pneumonitis, from chlamydia for example, and need to be treated systemically with erythromycin syrup in addition to topical therapy. Furthermore, the mother and her sexual partners need to be treated as well. Intravenous ceftriaxone should be instituted if one suspects *Neisseria gonorrhoeae*. Evaluation for disseminated gonococcal infection should be carefully assessed including blood and cerebrospinal fluid cultures, with appropriate antibiotic therapy of the infant.

Reference: Vander and Gault, pp. 72–5; Wilson, pp. 365–6; Cullom and Chang, pp. 197–200

71. Answer: C

Of all the options listed, this micro-organism is not among the common bacteria found associated with this entity.

Reference: Vander and Gault, pp. 72–5; Wilson, pp. 365–6; Cullom and Chang, pp. 197–200

72. Answer: C

This patient is severely hemodynamically compromised and the most appropriate action is immediate DC cardioversion. Digoxin, even when given intravenously, can take several hours to work. In some cases, there may be a role for anti-arrhythmics and β-blockers but this patient is severely compromised and immediate cardioversion is needed. Anticoagulation with heparin has a role in reducing embolic events in atrial fibrillation and may be considered once the acute episode has been dealt with.

Reference: Cummins, pp. 3.11–3.12

73. Answer: D

Atrial fibrillation can cause embolic stroke but embolic stroke is not a risk factor for atrial fibrillation. Thyrotoxicosis, mitral valve disease, coronary artery disease and excessive consumption of alcohol are all recognized causes of atrial fibrillation. Other causes include atrial septal defects, cardiomyopathy and recent cardiac surgery.

Reference: Kelley, pp. 416–17

74. Answer: B

The rhythm shown is ventricular tachycardia. Atropine would not be a suitable agent in this case as this increases the heart rate. All the other agents can be used in the management of this patient.

Reference: Cummins, pp. 1.17, 4.6

75. Answer: B

The recommended ACLS action is DC shock unsynchronized at 200 J and if unsuccessful in cardioversion, stepwise increments up to 360 J can be used. Intravenous epinephrine can be given after three shocks.

Reference: Cummins, pp. 1.17, 4.6

76. Answer: B

The adverse effects on the fetus of maternal phenylketonuria correlate with the degree of hyperphenylalaninemia and it is therefore recommended that a low phenylalanine diet is commenced prior to conception. Management of these patients should be supervised by physicians with special knowledge of this condition.

Reference: Bradley et al., p. 1599

77. Answer: C

Temporal arteritis must be excluded in this woman. She gives a history that includes headaches and scalp tenderness and also muscle aching and stiffness. Temporal arteritis is associated with polymyalgia rheumatica and her muscle aching is probably due to this. The most useful first investigation is an ESR. If the ESR is elevated, treatment with steroids should begin immediately followed by a temporal artery biopsy.

Reference: Rudy and Kurowski, p. 463

78. Answer: E

Endometrial cancer is associated with excessive estrogen stimulation of the endometrium. The exogenous or endogenous increase in a woman's estrogen levels can cause overstimulation of the endometrium and hence increase the risk of endometrial cancer. In obesity there is peripheral conversion of estrogen in fat cells. Other recognized factors include early menarche and late menopause, nulliparity and estrogen-secreting tumors. Ten per cent of women with endometrial cancer have diabetes and over 50% of all women with endometrial cancer have hypotension. There is no proven link with ischemic heart disease.

Reference: Symonds, p. 272

79. Answer: C

The workers most at risk of developing mesothelioma are auto workers involved with car brakes as they deal with asbestos, which is a known risk factor for mesothelioma. Unlike bronchial carcinoma, no association with smoking has been found.

Reference: Kelley, p. 2038

80. Answer: E

Renal agenesis is associated with oligohydramnios; all the others mentioned above are associated with poly-hydramnios. The fetus produces less urine, therefore causing oligohydramnios.

Reference: Symonds, p. 69

81. Answer: A

The most common heart defect is ventricular septal defect followed by patent ductus arteriosus and atrial septal defects.

Reference: Hull and Johnston, p. 135

82. Answer: A

The most common cause of spontaneous pneumothorax is the rupture of a small bleb at the apex of the lung. This condition is particularly common in thin young men and smokers.

Reference: Fauci et al., p. 1232

83. Answer: A

Human breast milk contains less sodium, potassium and chloride; if dehydration occurs the risk of hypernatremia is less. The presence of IgA, lysozymes, macrophages and lymphocytes provides immunological defense against disease in breast-fed infants.

Reference: Hull and Johnston, p. 77

84. Answer: D

Bereavement (also grief or mourning) describes a range of normal behaviors precipitated by the death of a loved one. This reaction may become the focus of clinical attention because its manifestations overlap with symptoms characteristic of major depressive disorder (MDD) (e.g. feelings of sadness, insomnia, poor appetite, weight loss, difficulty concentrating, irritability or tearfulness). Although most persons regard the sad mood as normal, they may seek medical help for the neurovegetative symptoms. The diagnosis of MDD is not given unless the symptoms are still present 2 months following the loss. In addition, the presence of symptoms atypical of normal bereavement may help in the diagnostic decision. These atypical features include inappropriate or excessive guilt, suicidal ideation or behavior, intense feelings or morbid preoccupation with worthlessness, marked psychomotor retardation or functional impairment, and hallucinations (other than transiently hearing the voice or seeing the image of the loved one).

Reference: DSM–IV, pp. 684–5

85. Answer: D

Defense mechanisms, also called coping styles, are automatic psychological processes (of which the individual is commonly unaware), that protect the individual against anxiety (as well as from the awareness of internal or external dangers or stressors) by mediating his or her reaction to emotional conflict and to stress. These mechanisms are divided into categories that DSM–IV calls 'defense levels'. The 'high adaptive level' mechanisms result in optimal adaptation in the handling of stressors by maximizing gratification and allowing and promoting optimum balance between conflicting motives. Examples of defenses at this level include sublimation, humor, altruism, anticipation, etc. Increasingly less high adaptive levels of defense include 'mental inhibitions' (e.g. repression, displacement); 'minor image distortions' (e.g. devaluation, idealization); 'disavowal' (e.g., denial, rationalization); 'major image distortions' (e.g. autistic fantasy, splitting); 'action' (e.g. acting out, withdrawal) and 'defensive dysregulation' (e.g. delusional projection, psychotic distortion).

Reference: DSM–IV, pp. 751–2

86. Answer: E

During middle childhood, interest in relationships with peers and teachers expands, and the ability to play games with rules and to develop friendships develops. However, the two sexes engage in fairly different kinds of activities and games. Boys tend to play in larger groups, and their play tends to be rougher and more expansive. They are more likely to interrupt each other, to refuse to comply with other boys' demands, heckle a speaker or call each other names. Girls, on the other hand, tend to form close, intimate friendships with one or two other girls, and these friendships are marked by the sharing of confidences. In all-girl groups, girls are more likely to

express agreement with what another speaker just said, to pause to allow other girl to speak, and to acknowledge somebody else's point.

Reference: Hales and Yudofsky, pp. 124–5

87. Answer: C

Many variables influence guaiac-based tests, including dietary factors like peroxidases and non-human hemoglobin; for this reason it is important to consider and modify diet when performing guaiac-based tests. Fecal rehydration markedly raises the sensitivity of guaiac-based tests but reduces specificity. Many believe that oral iron causes positive results on guaiac-based tests. Although the dark green or black appearance of iron in stools can be confused with the blue typical of a positive guaiac-based test, iron administered orally does not cause positive guaiac reactions. Antacids and antidiarrheal drugs containing bismuth also render the stool dark and may confound the reading of guaiac-based tests. There is an inconsistency of fecal occult blood tests in detecting fecal blood. Some of the tests require 10 mg per gram of stools (10 ml of daily blood loss) to be positive 50% of the time, but stools containing less than 1 mg/g can result in positive tests.

Reference: Rockey

88. Answer: E

The overwhelming risk factor for the development of esophageal adenocarcinoma is the progression of columnar epithelium to Barrett's metaplasia as a result of gastroesophageal reflux disorder. While smoking and alcohol use are significant risk factors for the development of squamous cell carcinoma of the esophagus, they are not important in the epidemiology of esophageal adenocarcinoma.

Reference: Greenfield, pp. 699–700

89. Answer: B

A parametric method requires that the distribution be known and that the data be normally distributed. Non-parametric methods make fewer assumptions regarding the shape of the distribution, and therefore may be useful when the shape of the distribution is unknown or in cases where there is a possibility that the distribution will have a non-standard shape. Non-parametric methods may also be used to provide an alternative to parametric methods and to confirm a suspected relationship.

Reference: Mould, p.108

90. Answer: D

Parametric tests rely on additional assumptions regarding a distribution, and they assume that it is meaningful to measure the actual differences between data values. Some parametric coefficients (such as the Pearson correlation coefficient) are considered to be more robust or sensitive than their non-parametric counterparts, but this does not universally hold true. Parametric tests, however, are not easier to integrate with regression, and are no more easily reproducible. Because they require a known distribution, they are actually more difficult to use with different types of data sets.

Reference: Hennekens *et al.*, pp. 102–3

91. Answer: A

The relative risk (RR) provides a measure of the risk of contracting a given injury, illness or state (here, head injury) in one group (exposed) versus another (unexposed). Because the RR refers to the risk of contracting a given state, it is clearly related to the incidence (rather than prevalence) of disease. The relative risk is calculated by dividing the incidence in the exposed group over the incidence in the unexposed group. It provides a measure of the relative chances of a patient having a given state (again, in this case, head injury) if they are exposed or unexposed to a given risk. If the incidence in both groups is the same, then the relative risk will be 1. The value of the relative risk is therefore not sensitive to the actual incidence in either of the groups, but instead to the relative incidence in the two groups. The risk difference, however (answer C), is sensitive to the actual incidences and not simply to the ratio. This has important clinical implications when reading a study, since a large relative risk with a very small risk difference may be statistically significant without being clinically significant. For example, if the relative risk of contracting Hashimoto encephalopathy (a rare encephalopathy) in milk drinkers versus non-milk drinkers is 3.2, but the risk difference is only 0.0003, then the relative risk, while large, still would not spur a campaign against drinking milk. Stated otherwise, if I had three times the amount of money that is currently in my wallet, I still would not have enough to buy a car.

Reference: Powell and Barber-Foss; Hennekens *et al.*, pp. 93–5

92. Answer: A

The RR cannot be calculated directly from a case-control study because patients in a case-control study are recruited based on their disease status rather than their exposure status. Therefore, the actual incidence cannot be calculated from a case-control study, and because the incidence is required to calculate the RR, the RR cannot be calculated directly. While the RR cannot be calculated directly, it can be closely approximated (in most cases) by the odds ratio. Therefore, when reading studies utilizing case-control designs, one should be suspicious of RR claims, especially if the study does not explicitly state that the RR is being approximated by utilizing the odds ratio.

Reference: Hennekens *et al.*, pp. 79–81

93. Answer: B

Since this study was conducted at what is obviously a specialized center, one would expect that their patients would have more severe disease than the majority of the population. Similarly, patients who attend such a specialized clinic are probably more motivated to be compliant, and therefore there is probably substantial selection bias in this study, which does not necessarily constitute a problem as long as it is addressed. While the other sources of bias are always of concern, they are of no more concern here than anywhere else.

94. Answer: C

Since this type of study involves following a cohort of patients across time, it is referred to as a cohort study. It is true that it is also a prospective study, but a cohort study is a type of prospective study and therefore would represent the more correct response. A clinical trial generally refers to a study where some intervention was undertaken, and usually refers to a randomized controlled trial. This clearly is not a case-control study, since patients were selected before there were any incident cases.

Reference: Hennekens *et al.*, pp. 153–77

95. Answer: D

Cohort studies are better equipped to aid in suggesting causality because they enrol patients at an early stage and follow them over time rather than taking patients who already have disease and looking back. There are also fewer concerns regarding control group selection. Cohort studies, because of the large number of patients that need to be studied and the long-term nature of the studies, are more expensive (and take much longer to complete) than case-control studies.

96. Answer: A

The *p* value, one of the most ubiquitous statistical terms in the medical literature, is also one of the most commonly misunderstood. It does not represent the probability that the effect itself is due to chance but rather the probability that the effect observed – or a more extreme one – could be due to chance alone.

Reference: Hennekens *et al.*, pp. 32–3

97. Answer: C

The cutoff of 0.05 for statistically significant *p* values is indeed an arbitrary one. Still, because the cutoff has been generally accepted, there cannot be any such thing as an almost statistically significant result; any *p* value above 0.05, regardless of by how much, is by definition no longer statistically significant. Clinical significance is more difficult to assess adequately from the information supplied, and must be decided given the clinical scenario under study. While it is possible, and even likely, that this *p* value represented a clinically significant relationship between leukoplakia and head and neck cancers, this cannot be determined from the information given. Therefore, C remains the best answer.

Reference: Rosner, pp. 551–84

98. Answer: A

Because patients switch between two treatment methods after set periods of time, this would best be described as a crossover study. In this type of study, patients serve as their own controls, thus decreasing both the cost of the study and the time needed for follow-up, as well as providing ideal controls.

Reference: Hennekens *et al.*, pp. 178–212

99. Answer: D

Crossover studies assume that an effect will be visible relatively quickly (i.e. in this case a reduction in episodes of otitis media) since otherwise it would be unclear whether or not an effect was due to one or the other intervention. They also assume there will be no residual effect since again, it would otherwise be impossible to determine which intervention was responsible for which effect. Likewise, a washout period is often included between the different interventions in order to minimize the problems associated with the effect of one intervention becoming evident only once the other intervention has begun.

Reference: Hennekens *et al.*, pp. 272–86

TEST TWO

Satellite health center

1. You manage a 15-year-old girl with severe asthma, who has been hospitalized over 20 times. Her current regimen includes albuterol metered dose inhalers (MDIs), ipratropium bromide MDIs and daily oral steroids. She has done well on this regimen and has not required hospitalization in over 3 months. She comes to your office today and informs you that a home pregnancy test was positive. You repeat a urine pregnancy test, confirming the pregnancy. Your counseling includes discussing the following:

A. abortion should be considered because she is only a child herself
B. abortion should be considered because the pregnancy will exacerbate her asthma
C. abortion should be considered because of the medications she has been taking
D. corticosteroids, albuterol and ipratropium bromide are not known to be teratogenic agents
E. she is not at increased risk for spontaneous abortion secondary to her asthma

2. A 5-day-old is brought to your clinic, as the mother is concerned about a bruise on the face. The birth history reveals that the birth was a vaginal delivery with the assistance of forceps. Physical examination reveals a well-circumscribed, firm nodule the size of a nickel with purplish discoloration on the right cheek. The most appropriate next step is to:

A. refer to a plastic surgeon
B. offer reassurance to the mother that this is normal and will resolve spontaneously
C. obtain a skull radiograph
D. refer them to a geneticist for screening and counseling
E. obtain a biopsy

3. You see a 32-year-old teacher in your clinic who is complaining of an 8-month history of chronic diarrhea, abdominal distension and weight loss. The diagnosis of lactose intolerance was made and she started a lactose-free diet without significant improvement in her symptoms. Sudan stain of her stool was reported as positive. You referred her for a jejunal biopsy that revealed atrophic mucosa with blunting and flattening of the villi, and the valvulae conniventes exhibited a distinctive scalloped appearance. Which of the following results best supports your diagnosis?

A. positive antigliadin antibodies
B. positive antiendomysial antibodies
C. positive antireticulin antibodies
D. all of the above

4. A 60-year-old patient presents to your office complaining of a painful swollen left knee. The swelling started 1 day ago and was associated with fever of 101°F. On physical examination the knee is swollen, erythematous and tender. Active and passive range of motion is limited. Which of the following results obtained on synovial fluid analysis would not support the diagnosis of gout (monosodium urate disease)?

A. white blood cell count of 24 000 cells/μl
B. weak positive birefringence in polarized light
C. when a red plate compensator is used the crystals appear yellow when parallel and blue when perpendicular to the axis of the compensator
D. needle-shaped crystals

5. Anxious parents come to the clinic with their 2-year-old child. They live in an old building and are concerned about lead exposure. The organ systems most affected by lead poisoning include all of the following except:

A. central nervous system
B. liver
C. peripheral nervous system
D. kidney
E. bone marrow

6. You see a 3-year-old Chinese child for the first time at the clinic and you suspect that the child has trisomy 21. The family are recent immigrants to the USA. Key features of trisomy 21 (Down syndrome) include all of the following except:

A. macrocephaly
B. hypotonia
C. short neck
D. congenital heart disease
E. short stature

7.   A 45-year-old professor presents with a droopy lid, decreased sweat and a small pupil, all on the left side. With dim illumination there is no change in the appearance of the pupil. All of the following regarding this entity are appropriate except:

A.   confirm the diagnosis with a cocaine test
B.   obtain a chest X-ray of the lung or CT scan of the chest
C.   obtain carotid angiogram
D.   inquire of any history of previous neck, thoracic or thyroid surgery
E.   rule out a cranial nerve palsy

8.   An adolescent female comes to your clinic for her yearly school physical. In evaluating her pubertal development you find that her breasts are elevated with areola enlargement, and her pubic hair is dark, coarse, curly and sparsely covers the pubes. She is Tanner developmental stage:

A.   stage I
B.   stage II
C.   stage III
D.   stage IV
E.   stage V

9.   A 65-year-old male patient comes in for a routine check-up. On cardiac examination of the patient, you hear a mid-systolic ejection murmur. Which of the following conditions would NOT explain this finding:

A.   aortic stenosis or aortic sclerosis
B.   hypertrophic obstructive cardiomyopathy
C.   coarctation of the aorta
D.   ventricular septal defect (VSD) with a left-to-right shunt
E.   congenital bicuspid valve

10.   A 72-year-old Vietnamese woman presents with a history of chills and fevers for the last 3 days. She also has a chronic cough productive of yellowish sputum. Her past medical history is significant for asthma which was diagnosed 3 months ago, left lower lobe pneumonia 1 month ago and chronic diarrhea. Review of systems is positive for weight loss of 3 lb over the last year and occasional hot flashes. She is a non-smoker. On physical examination she has a blood pressure of 100/80, respiratory rate of 24, heart rate of 80 per minute and oxygen saturation on room air of 94%. Examination of her chest reveals crackles over her left lower lung fields. The rest of the exam is normal. Bronchoscopy reveals an endobronchial tumor. All of the following are true about this patient except:

A.   biopsy of this tumor carries a risk of profuse bleeding
B.   imaging of the liver will probably reveal metastatic disease
C.   presence of a paraneoplastic syndrome would support the diagnosis
D.   treatment of choice is surgical excision
E.   24-hour urine collection will probably reveal an increased vanillylmandelic acid level

Office

11.   All of the following are acceptable alternative treatments in patients with sulfonamide allergy who are diagnosed with *Pneumocystis carinii* pneumonia (PCP), except:

A.   aerosolized pentamidine
B.   dapsone + trimethoprim
C.   atovaquone
D.   trimetrexate + folinic acid
E.   clindamycin + primaquine

12.   A young theater student comes to your office complaining of 'nerves'. He reports that he can play his parts without difficulty during rehearsals, but when he is getting ready for a performance his heart pounds, his hands sweat and tremble and he feels lightheaded and nauseated. He reports that in spite of having an excellent memory and being able to learn his parts readily, he is afraid that he will not remember a line and will embarrass himself on stage. Recently the symptoms have become so bad that he did not show up for performance on two occasions, and he is now afraid that he will have to drop out of the college theater group. The most likely diagnosis is:

A.   panic disorder with agoraphobia
B.   generalized anxiety disorder
C.   avoidant personality disorder
D.   somatization disorder
E.   social phobia

13.   A 34-year-old white female presents in your office with the complaint of several episodes of blurred vision lasting 15–20 minutes with zigzag visual disturbances preceding a unilateral headache accompanied by nausea and vomiting. She gives a positive family history in her mother and maternal aunt including car-sickness as a child. All of the following can precipitate this patient's complaint except:

A.   amitriptyline
B.   aged cheeses
C.   chocolate
D.   wine
E.   birth control pills

14. An obese 45-year-old black female is seen in your office and noted to have bilateral swollen, hyperemic optic discs. All of the following may be associated with this presentation except:

A. severe loss of central visual acuity
B. transient visual loss lasting seconds
C. double vision
D. headache
E. enlarged ventricles on CT scan

15. A 6-year-old boy is brought to your office with coughing and low-grade fever. On physical examination he has crackles localized in his left lower lung fields on auscultation. A chest radiograph confirms left lingular infiltrate. You diagnose bacterial pneumonia. You know the family well and the child has no symptoms of respiratory distress. The antibiotic contraindicated in this age group is:

A. erythromycin
B. trimethoprim–sulfamethoxizole
C. amoxicillin with clavulanic acid
D. ciprofloxacin
E. cephalexin

16. A 3-week-old infant, known to have cystic fibrosis, is seen in your office with a fever, increased respiratory effort and crackles in the left lung. The organism most probably responsible for the child's pneumonia is:

A. *Pseudomonas aeruginosa*
B. *Klebsiella pneumoniae*
C. *Mycobacterium avium*
D. *Aspergillus*
E. *Staphylococcus aureus*

17. A 17-year-old girl comes to your office, alone. She is concerned, as she has skipped two menstrual periods. A urine pregnancy test is positive and your bimanual examination reveals an enlarged uterus, estimated to be 6 weeks pregnant. She asks you not to call her parents. The next step in management is to:

A. inform her of the medical options and have her make an appointment when she decides
B. explain to her the medical issues and then discuss her reluctance to talk with her parents
C. tell her you are legally obligated to talk with her parents
D. refer her to an obstetrician
E. tell her you understand her concerns, and that she has a week to tell her parents before you do

18. 'Shaken baby' syndrome is an unfortunately common form of non-accidental trauma in children under 6 months of age. Of the following findings, the pathognomonic one is:

A. subdural hematoma
B. cerebral edema
C. posterior rib fractures
D. finger impression bruises on rib cage
E. retinal hemorrhages

19. A previously well 35-year-old African-American male with HIV diagnosed 5 years ago with a CD4 count of 150 comes to your office complaining of severe shortness of breath on exertion for the last few days. You saw the patient a few weeks ago when you started him on anti-retroviral medication and *Pneumocystis carinii* pneumonia (PCP) prophylaxis. His physical exam is significant for blood pressure of 100/70, pulse rate of 100 per minute and respiratory rate of 20. His physical exam is significant for pale mucosae. No lymph nodes are palpable. Heart sounds are normal; he has a regular rate and rhythm but is tachycardic. The rest of the exam is normal. His hemoglobin is 8.0 mg/dl, hematocrit is 27% and reticulocytes are 6.7. His peripheral smear shows 'bite' cells. Coombs test is negative. The leukocyte alkaline phosphatase is normal.

The most likely diagnosis for this patient's anemia is:

A. autoimmune hemolytic anemia
B. paroxysmal nocturnal hemoglobinuria
C. lymphoproliferative disease
D. pyruvate kinase deficiency
E. glucose-6-phosphate dehydrogenase (G6PD) deficiency

20. A 58-year-old white male presents to your office noting drooping of his lids and onset of double vision in the early afternoon. He relates resolution of his symptoms following his naps with recurrence later in the evening. To establish your diagnosis, you should:

A. obtain an MRI to rule out a brain stem lesion
B. administer edrophonium chloride
C. send off thyroid function tests
D. assess the patient's cranial nerves, 3, 4 and 6 in particular
E. reassure the patient and check for any vitamin deficiency

21. A 45-year-old white female presents to your office with a complaint of awakening with a bad headache and diplopia. You notice that she is unable to look up, down or in with her

left eye. This is accompanied by a droopy lid. Pupillary exam reveals a mid-dilated pupil on the same side. You should immediately:

A. admit the patient and obtain an MRI/MRA
B. evaluate the fundus for disc edema to assess evidence for hydrocephalus
C. obtain orbital films to rule out a possible fracture with ocular muscle entrapment
D. suspect Adie's tonic pupil and assess reflexes
E. rule out pharmacologic pupillary dilation

22.   Fragile X syndrome is the most common form of mental retardation in males. The following are all characteristic of the syndrome except:

A. micro-orchidism
B. hyperactivity
C. long face
D. protruding, wide ears
E. high arched palate

23.   A 13-year-old boy is brought to your office with nausea and vomiting. His parents say it started only 2 hours ago, but the vomiting has been so frequent they are concerned. The boy complains of acute lower abdominal pain and intermittently grabs at his pants. On physical examination his abdomen is unremarkable, but his left testis is enlarged and very tender to palpation. The next step in management is:

A. initiate oral antibiotic therapy
B. reassure the parents and see the child in follow up in 1–2 days
C. attempt to detorsion the testicle
D. prompt pediatric surgical consultation
E. ultrasound of the scrotum

24.   A 70-year-old man comes to your clinic complaining of generalized weakness, weight loss and difficulty walking. He has seen a number of doctors and even a complementary medicine therapist without any diagnosis being made. Over the last 2 weeks he has had difficulty swallowing. On examination you find a cachectic elderly male with mild impairment of palatal elevation. He has brisk reflexes in the legs and bilateral extensor planter responses. In the upper limbs he has marked fasciculations but absent reflexes. There are no cognitive changes. The most likely diagnosis is:

A. amyotrophic lateral sclerosis (ALS)
B. Guillain–Barré syndrome
C. Creutzfeldt–Jakob disease
D. myasthenia gravis

25.   Which of the following drugs can slow the progression of amyotrophic lateral sclerosis (ALS)?

A. riluzole
B. aspirin
C. clopidogrel
D. brain-derived neurotrophic factor (BDNF)

26–28.   A 25-year-old woman presents with a 3-month history of blurred vision at the end of the day. However, over the last 2 days she has had dysuria and was prescribed ampicillin by her primary care physician for a urinary tract infection. She now presents to the ER with increasing weakness more marked axially and difficulty swallowing and breathing. On examination she has bilateral ptosis, ophthalmoplegia, and proximal muscle weakness. Her reflexes are brisk initially but diminish with repetitive stimulation.

26.   The likely diagnosis is:

A. myasthenia gravis (MG)
B. amyotrophic lateral sclerosis (ALS)
C. depression
D. Eaton–Lambert syndrome

27.   If myasthenia is suspected, which of the following investigations will be least likely to help in making the diagnosis:

A. EMG
B. anti-acetylcholine receptor antibodies
C. CT of thorax
D. MRI of brain

28.   The following are useful in the treatment of myasthenia gravis (MG) except:

A. steroids
B. pyridostigmine
C. thymectomy
D. azathioprine
E. aminoglycosides

29.   Your patient is a 66-year-old male who first came to your office 1 month ago for the workup of painless rectal bleeding. His medical history is notable for chronic obstetric pulmonary disease (COPD) due to a 50 cigarette per day smoking history, renal insufficiency (creatinine 2.2 mg/dl), and he is an admitted alcoholic who drinks 10–12 drinks per evening. At the time of the first visit, you referred the patient for a colonoscopy, and a blood sample was sent for testing for carcinoembryonic antigen (CEA). The

colonoscopy shows an annular lesion in the proximal recto-sigmoid, and the biopsy specimen reveals adenocarcinoma. The CEA is elevated. Which of the following is FALSE regarding the interpretation of CEA in this context?

A. CEA is a useful screening tool, and can help early diagnosis of colorectal CA
B. CEA is useful as a prognostic indicator
C. CEA is useful in detecting tumor recurrence post-operatively
D. CEA can be used to direct follow-up surgical intervention
E. CEA is elevated in a number of benign conditions, including COPD, pancreatitis and renal failure

30. A 33-year-old male is seen by your office for evaluation of a chest X-ray showing a small (1.5 cm) lesion in the periphery of his right middle lung field. The radiograph was obtained after a sports injury in which it was thought he may have suffered a rib fracture. He is a non-smoker (and always has been), with no family history of lung cancer. There is no evidence of current or recent infection, and he denies any constitutional symptoms. Which of the following would be the most appropriate next step in the workup of this pulmonary nodule?

A. obtaining any previous chest radiographs
B. CT-guided biopsy
C. video thoracoscopy and wedge biopsy
D. no further workup is necessary

31. The older brother of the patient in the previous question decides that he should obtain a chest radiograph, and it shows a small (2 cm) lesion in the central region of his right upper lung field. A chest X-ray from 8 years ago shows no evidence of the lesion. He is 51 years old, and has a 20 cig-arette per day history of smoking. A CT scan is performed, which demonstrates suspicious morphology of the solitary nodule, and no other findings. He elects to have a right upper lobectomy performed, and a tissue diagnosis of squamous cell carcinoma (SCC) is made. Which of the following is FALSE regarding this type of cancer?

A. SCCs in the lung usually arise centrally
B. smoking and radon are both risk factors for SCC
C. survival is better than for small cell carcinoma
D. it is the most common type of lung cancer in women

32. A patient presents to your office in the second trimester and asks you whether or not ingesting monosodium glutamate may be dangerous to the health of her fetus. You recall seeing a reference to the fact that many of the studies regarding the teratogenicity of common products have been 'under-powered'. The power of a study may be increased by:

A. increasing the sample size
B. an increased proportion of patients with the event
C. well matched controls
D. A and B
E. A and C

33. Regarding patients with AIDS and CMV infection:

A. CMV retinitis is the most common retinal infection
B. infection usually occurs with CD4 counts < 50 cells/μl
C. infection requires induction therapy with either ganciclovir or foscarnet
D. all of the above
E. none of the above

34. A 28-year-old woman presents to your office concerned that she may have contracted HIV from a recent sexual escapade. She is interested in being tested for the HIV virus, and asks you about the different tests that are available for detecting HIV. You explain to the patient that a test for a virus such as HIV should:

A. be highly specific and sensitive
B. be highly sensitive only
C. have a low false positive rate only
D. have a lot of power
E. none of the above

Emergency room

35. A 35-year-old prostitute presents with an acute vesicular skin rash involving the left side of the face in a trigeminal-nerve distribution. All of the following pertain to this patient except:

A. this entity may be the first clinical manifestation of HIV infection
B. initiate systemic therapy with aciclovir
C. it is highly contagious to those with a negative history of chicken pox
D. if HIV-positive, the patient is at risk for CMV retinopathy, the second most common ocular infection in AIDS
E. there is a good chance of ocular involvement if the V1 branch is affected

36. A 55-year-old engineer who has been a lifelong smoker is admitted to the ER having had a grand mal seizure at work. On further questioning he admits to increasingly frequent headaches for the last 2–3 months and difficulty concentrating at work. He has been off his food and reports 8 lb weight loss. His wife also noted a change in his behavior

during the same period of time. These findings would be most consistent with the diagnosis of:

A. primary or secondary brain tumor
B. migraine
C. cluster headaches
D. tension headaches

37. A 24-year-old man has been involved in a road traffic accident and has sustained multiple injuries. The first priority in the management of this patient when he arrives in the emergency room is:

A. insertion of an intravenous catheter
B. administration of oxygen
C. assessing the airway
D. checking blood pressure
E. checking oxygen saturation

38. A 24-year-old diabetic college student presents with a red eye, blurred vision, fever, headache and double vision. On examination, you find eyelid edema, tenderness and restricted ocular motility of the left eye on attempted eye movement. The patient relates having a dental infection a month previously that was treated with broad-spectrum antibiotics. To ascertain your diagnosis, you should:

A. obtain blood cultures and lumbar puncture
B. check for an afferent pupillary defect
C. obtain a finger stick to assess the blood sugar and evaluate the nasal mucosa and palate
D. obtain CT scan of the orbit and sinuses
E. all of the above

39. A healthy 6-year-old child presents to the ER with evidence of a rapidly growing lesion in the left eye over 72 hours with marked eyelid edema and a palpable mass noted superiorly. There is marked downward displacement of the globe. A CT scan reveals bony destruction with a mass noted in the superior orbit. The most likely diagnosis is:

A. retinoblastoma
B. leukemia
C. metastatic neuroblastoma
D. rhabdomyosarcoma
E. teratoma

40. You are asked to evaluate a patient involved in a brawl and found to have a possible blowout fracture of the right eye. All of the following are true regarding this condition except:

A. double vision
B. hypesthesia of the ipsilateral cheek and upper lip
C. restricted eye movement
D. crepitus (subcutaneous emphysema) on palpation of the eyelids
E. emergent orbital decompression to correct double vision

41. A local gangster is brought into the ER after a shoot-out in which he sustained a gunshot wound to the face and left eye. All of the following are appropriate measurements except:

A. protect the eye with a shield
B. administer a tetanus toxoid
C. obtain an MRI of orbits and brain to rule out a foreign body
D. make the patient n.p.o. for immediate surgery
E. initiate broad spectrum systemic antibiotics

42. A 33-year-old woman is brought by EMS to the ER with convulsions. On arrival, she has her eyes tightly shut and resists attempts to open them, shakes her head from side to side, intermittently screams single words, and her limbs exhibit flailing movements without synchrony. During the convulsion, she does not follow commands, but localizes with her right hand to sternal rubbing. After 1 minute of this spell, she wakes up and is oriented and alert, but fatigued, and says that she does not remember getting to the ER. Review of her large medical records reveals numerous visits to the ER with a great variety of complaints including severe headaches, as well as numerous hospital admissions spanning several years, including workups for irritable bowel disease, chest pain and palpitations, RLQ pain, dysmenorrhea and multiple joint pains. All the prior examinations, including repeated laboratory tests, imaging studies, and invasive diagnostic procedures (including two laparotomies) have been fruitless. The most likely diagnosis is:

A. borderline personality disorder
B. malingering
C. somatization disorder
D. hypochondriasis
E. epilepsy

43. A 12-year-old girl comes to the ER complaining of a sore, swollen right knee. Additional history reveals that she has intermittently had abdominal pain and an erythematous rash, although neither is present at this time. Over the past 24 hours her right knee has started to swell, and has become stiff, red and tender. On physical examination she has no rash, her knee is hot and erythematous, and a large effusion is present. The most appropriate management at this time is:

A. obtain a rheumatoid factor
B. obtain a nuclear medicine bone scan
C. obtain radiographs of the joint
D. obtain an antinuclear antibody titer
E. aspirate the joint

44. A 15-year-old with chronic sinusitis presents in the ER complaining of blurred vision and swelling of the right eye. On examination the right infraorbital and supraorbital eyelids are markedly swollen, tender and indurated. You are concerned that he has mild proptosis. The first test to perform is:

A. white blood cell count with differential
B. blood culture
C. CT scan of head
D. lumbar puncture
E. eye/conjunctiva culture

45. An 18-month-old is brought into the ER with scalded skin on the buttocks and heels of the feet. The mother says 'the child crawled into the bath tub and turned the hot water on'. Non-accidental trauma is suspected. Appropriate management includes all of the following except:

A. referral to child protective services
B. radiographic skeletal survey
C. referral to Department of Social Services
D. confrontation of accompanying parent
E. review of medical records at all local hospitals

46. A 45-year-old patient is brought to the ER by her family because of fever and confusion. She started feeling unwell 4 days ago, started having fever and chills and was increasingly short of breath with minimal exertion.

On physical examination the patient has a pulse rate of 100, blood pressure of 98/70, respiratory rate of 24 and a temperature of 101.3. The patient does not seem to be in apparent distress but is obtunded. She looks pale and mildly jaundiced. Examination of the heart, lungs and abdomen is unremarkable. She has no focal neurological deficit. Creatine kinase and electrolytes are normal.

Labs:
Hematocrit   26%
WBC   6400/μl (normal differential)
Platelets   6000/μl
Creatinine   6.4 mg/dl
BUN   75 mg/dl
LDH   1700

All of the following would support your diagnosis of thrombotic thrombocytopenic purpura (TTP) except:

A. normal Coombs test
B. peripheral smear showing fragmented RBCs
C. abnormal coagulation studies
D. urinalysis showing proteinuria
E. normal lumbar puncture

47. Your patient is a 19-year-old male who has presented to the ER with localizing RLQ pain, anorexia, and a WBC of 12.5×10^9/l. The pain has become increasingly focal over the last 4–5 hours, and your suspicion of appendicitis is high enough to warrant a trip to the OR without confirmatory radiologic exam. What is the most appropriate perioperative antibiotic for this patient?

A. cefazolin
B. ampicillin, gentamicin, metronidazole
C. single dose cefotetan
D. single dose cefoxitin

48. You are a junior surgical resident cross-covering the pediatric ER, and you are called to evaluate a 2-month-old male infant. He is brought in by an anxious mother who recently noticed a new bulge in the baby's left groin, as well as colicky behavior and decreased interest in food. On your exam, you notice a non-reducible bulge in the superior portion of the infant's left testicle, with no associated redness or tenderness. The baby has no known history of recent viral or other infections. Which of the following is TRUE regarding hernias in a pediatric population?

A. hernias in this age group are more commonly left-sided
B. many cases can be managed conservatively
C. recurrence of the hernia is less common than in the adult population
D. none of the above is true

49. A 22-year-old male farm worker is seen by you in the ER for a workplace injury (caused by a razor-wire fence) that occurred 12 hours ago, resulting in a laceration to his right outer shoulder. The laceration is approximately 3 cm long, through dermis, and at several points a small amount of adipose tissue can be seen at the base of the wound. The wound is otherwise clean, and the patient has received a dose of tetanus toxoid. Which of the following best describes the appropriate surgical technique for optimal cosmetic outcome?

A. skin should be closed with more tissue at deeper layers to cause wound eversion
B. skin should be closed with less tissue at deeper layers to cause wound inversion
C. skin should be closed flat to cause neither inversion nor eversion
D. after 12 hours the wound should not be closed primarily

50. You are called to see a 22-year-old male college student in the ER for a rule-out of appendicitis. As you are walking to the patient's room, one of the residents in the ER approaches you and says, 'It looks like an appy, but it doesn't

have all of the usual signs and symptoms... I'm curious to see what you think...' Which of the following statements about the manifestation and diagnosis of appendicitis is false?

A. virtually all patients present with pain and anorexia
B. fever is usually present
C. a non-operative approach is feasible
D. a positive family history is considered a risk factor for appendicitis
E. all of the above are true

Hospital

51. A 35-year-old male trauma patient is in the surgical intensive care unit (SICU), after having received multiple gunshot wounds to his pelvis, abdomen and chest. During his resuscitation, a splenectomy and lower lobectomy of his left lung were performed, as well as a small bowel resection and cystoplasty. He is now post-operative day 2 and still has a left chest tube in place, which has put out 400 cc of sanguinous fluid in the last 8 hours (150 cc in the previous 24 hours). He has some new onset bleeding from surgical incision sites. Coagulation studies are sent, and the PT INR is 2.4. Which of the following laboratory values correlates best with the severity of the patient's bleeding diathesis:

A. fibrinogen
B. d-dimer
C. fibrinogen degradation product (FDP)
D. PT/PTT
E. platelet count

52. Which of the following statements is FALSE regarding hernias in the adult population?

A. the majority of hernias occur in the inguinal region
B. indirect inguinal hernias are more common than direct inguinal hernias
C. 25% of males will develop inguinal hernias in their lifetime
D. femoral hernias are the most common type of hernia in women

53. You are evaluating a 63-year-old male with cirrhosis and end-stage liver disease (ESLD) as a possible candidate for a shunting procedure. Which of the following laboratory and clinical indicators is not considered highly predictive of the patient's perioperative mortality?

A. serum albumin
B. serum bilirubin
C. degree of encephalopathy
D. serum SGOT

54. While obtaining a brief medical history on the above patient, he tells you that he once had a very bad asthmatic hypersensitivity reaction to a local anesthetic that he remembers very well. 'Procaine – that's what it was. I'm 100% sure.' His wife confirms this recollection. Which of the following statements is TRUE regarding your choice of local anesthetics for this patient?

A. it is unlikely that this was a true hypersensitivity reaction – more likely a toxic side-effect
B. lidocaine would be an acceptable alternative for this patient
C. tetracaine would be an acceptable alternative for this patient
D. use of any local anesthetic should be avoided in this patient

55. A 42-year-old male with no significant past medical history is post-operative day 5 after an upper lobectomy procedure of his right lung. He remains intubated and has been persistently hypotensive (systolic BP 80–96, diastolic 50–60) and tachycardic (HR 105–115), with little improvement after repeated fluid boluses. Urine output has been 20–25 cc/h. His pre-operative vitals were 130/90 with a HR 70. His temperature is 102.4°F, and he has been febrile throughout most of his recovery, but blood cultures have been persistently negative. He is moderately sedated, but able to communicate that he has significant abdominal discomfort. His labs today are:

Na$^+$	130 mmol/l
BUN	22 mg/dl
WBC	8.7×10^9/l
K$^+$	6.0 mmol/l
Creatinine	1.7 mg/dl
Hemoglobin	11.3 g/dl
Cl$^-$	99 mmol/l
Glucose	72 mg/dl
Platelets	250×10^9/l
HCO$_3$	24 mmol/l

A brief trial of dopamine at doses up to 8 μg/kg had little effect on his blood pressure, and no change in his urine output. What is an appropriate therapeutic intervention to address his primary problem at this point?

A. dexamethasone IV
B. dialysis
C. dobutamine
D. free water restriction

56. Your patient is a 31-year-old female, recently diagnosed with myasthenia gravis (MG). She has invested a significant amount of time and energy researching the possible types

of treatment for her condition. She now comes to you for advice about whether or not to have a thymectomy performed. Which of the following is FALSE about thymectomy for patients with MG?

A. most patients with MG have an underlying thymoma
B. most patients with thymomas either have or will develop MG
C. thymomas are associated with other paraneoplastic syndromes, including red cell aplasia, Cushing syndrome, and hypogammaglobulinemia
D. thymectomy generally improves the symptoms of MG in this type of patient

57. A 68-year-old female is an unrestrained driver involved in a head-on motor vehicle crash at moderate speed. She struck the steering wheel forcibly with her chest, and is brought in to your trauma bay with significant chest pain, but otherwise stable. Her vitals are:

Temperature	97.8°F
BP	95/55 mmHg
HR	120/min
RR	18/min

On primary survey, she has bilateral breath sounds that are equal and clear, with no tracheal deviation. The force of the blow and the obvious tissue injury from the steering wheel makes you worry about the possibility of a traumatic aortic injury. Anteroposterior and lateral chest films are performed, and there are some disturbing findings. Which of the following is not considered a cardinal radiologic finding suggestive of possible aortic injury?

A. widened mediastinum
B. apical pleural capping
C. loss of aortic knob
D. obliteration of space between PA and aorta
E. all of the above are cardinal findings

58. Your patient is a 54-year-old male with a recently established diagnosis of mitral valve endocarditis. He has been experiencing some new symptoms of congestive heart failure including shortness of breath and dyspnea on exertion, as well as constitutional symptoms of fever, malaise and insomnia. Prior to initiation of a course of outpatient antibiotics, his physician requested a consultation from a cardiac surgeon to evaluate him. Which of the following is NOT a major criterion for surgery for infective endocarditis?

A. progressive heart failure
B. multiple embolic episodes
C. fungal endocarditis
D. development of heart block
E. all of the above are major criteria

59. A 63-year-old male patient of yours undergoes trans-esophageal echocardiography (TEE) to rule out intracardiac thrombus prior to undergoing semi-elective cardioversion for symptomatic atrial fibrillation. The study notes that he has moderate to severe aortic stenosis, but the patient denies any symptoms of angina, syncope or dyspnea. Which of the following are possible indications for aortic valve surgery in an asymptomatic patient?

A. aortic valve area $< 0.8\,cm^2$
B. mean systolic gradient > 50 mmHg
C. flow velocity across aortic valve > 4 m/s
D. all of the above are possible indications
E. surgery is not indicated in the asymptomatic patient

60. You perform a paracentesis in a patient with a known diagnosis of pyogenic peritonitis. Which of the results of the peritoneal fluid analysis would be unusual for your diagnosis?

A. gross appearance of the peritoneal fluid is turbid
B. protein concentration is > 2.5 g/dl
C. serum–ascites albumin gradient (SAG) is > 1.1 g/dl
D. cell count reveals predominantly polymorphonuclear leukocytes
E. the Gram stain is positive for presence of bacteria

61. What is the recommended workup of patients with malignant melanoma of less than 0.76 mm?

A. complete history and physical examination is acceptable as risk of metastasizing is low
B. sentinel node mapping should be performed
C. perform CT scan of head and abdomen
D. perform CBC and LFT

62. All of the following statements about treatment for breast cancer with tamoxifen are true, except:

A. antitumor effects of tamoxifen are thought to be due to its antiestrogenic activity, mediated by competitive inhibition of estrogen binding to estrogen receptors
B. owing to its antiestrogenic effect it reduces the risk of endometrial cancer
C. tamoxifen is indicated in pre- and postmenopausal women who have estrogen receptor-positive invasive breast cancer
D. in women treated for 5 years with tamoxifen there is a 50% annual reduction in recurrence rate and a 28% annual reduction in death rate
E. tamoxifen is used in the treatment of men with breast cancer

63. You are asked to consult on a 49-year-old male who, during a CT scan for abdominal trauma, is noted to have a

centrally located 1.5 × 1.5 cm lesion in the right lobe of his liver. He has a known 7-year history of chronic hepatitis B infection. Which of the following statements is FALSE regarding hepatocellular carcinoma (HCC)?

A. there is an association between HCC and hepatitis C virus (HCV) infection, but not hepatitis A virus (HAV) infection
B. most patients with HCC have an elevated AFP
C. HBsAg positivity yields over a 200-fold increased risk for HCC
D. this patient would not be eligible for liver transplant

64. Your patient is a 17-month-old female infant with trisomy 21 who is undergoing a Nissen fundoplication (for gastroesophageal reflux disorder) and pyloromyotomy (for gastric outlet obstruction). At surgery, the patient is discovered to have a previously undetected midgut malrotation. Which of the following is FALSE regarding the surgical management of this condition?

A. the cecum should be surgically fixated to the LUQ
B. the duodenum should be surgically fixated to the RLQ
C. the appendix should be removed
D. the malrotation should be rotated in a clockwise direction (surgeon's view) to relieve the malrotation
E. all of the above are true

65. You are managing the fluids for a 70-kg 63-year-old male who is postoperative day 3 after a sigmoidectomy for colonic adenocarcinoma. The patient is receiving D5 1/2 normal saline at a rate of 125 cc/h. Which of the following is the number of kcal/l of this intravenous fluid mixture?

A. 100 kcal/l
B. 135 kcal/l
C. 170 kcal/l
D. 205 kcal/l
E. none of the above

66. A patient is referred to your office for evaluation of chronic abdominal pain, and perioral paresthesias. You suspect that her symptoms are due to hypercalcemia and go on to conduct a history and physical exam to add weight to your suspicion. Which of the following physical exam findings is NOT consistent with a patient who is hypercalcemic?

A. hyperreflexia
B. abdominal pain
C. mental status changes
D. hypertension
E. all of the above are characteristic findings of hypercalcemia

67. After a thorough workup, the patient in question 66 is found to have an elevated parathyroid hormone level and no metabolic causes for her hypercalcemia. She is taken to the operating room for neck exploration and removal of pathologic parathyroid tissue. What are the most likely histopathologic findings for the procedure and the tissue removed?

A. pathologic findings in one gland
B. pathologic findings in two glands
C. pathologic findings in three glands
D. pathologic findings in all four glands

68. A 13-year-old boy had a viral illness 10 days ago and now presents with difficulty walking. Examination reveals generalized weakness of the face and limbs. The reflexes are absent. The most likely diagnosis is:

A. Guillain–Barré syndrome
B. amyotrophic lateral sclerosis
C. myasthenia gravis
D. Eaton–Lambert syndrome

69. Which of the following have been found to be useful in the management of Guillain–Barré syndrome (GBS):

A. plasmapheresis and intravenous immunoglobulins
B. steroids
C. cyclophosphamide
D. methotrexate

70. Hypotension as a result of verapamil administration may be treated with the use of which of the following agents?

A. procainamide
B. atropine
C. calcium chloride
D. bretylium tosylate
E. amiodarone

Other encounters

71. The following are true about Rinne's test except:

A. in pure sensorineural hearing loss, air conduction will be better than bone conduction
B. a Rinne's test is positive if bone is better than air
C. if the tympanic membrane is perforated or if the ossicles are disrupted, bone conduction will be better than air
D. if air conduction is better than bone then there may be no loss (normal), conductive, sensorineural or mixed
E. a tuning fork of frequency of 512 Hz is used

72. Recurrent panic attacks are most frequently caused by:

A. chronic obstructive pulmonary disease (COPD)
B. brain tumors, especially near the third ventricle
C. shift in sleep schedule
D. irritable bowel syndrome
E. psychoactive substance intoxication or withdrawal

73. Cataplexy is a manifestation of:

A. catatonia
B. periodic paralysis
C. akinetic epilepsy
D. narcolepsy
E. dissociative disorder

74. Causes of conduction loss include all the following except:

A. aminoglycosides
B. perforated or immobilized ear drum
C. wax
D. otosclerosis

75. The following are all true about Weber's test except:

A. in bilateral conduction hearing loss the sound is heard the same in both ears
B. in unilateral conduction hearing loss the sound is lateralized to the bad ear
C. in unilateral sensorineural hearing loss the sound is lateralized to the good ear
D. in unilateral sensorineural hearing loss the sound is lateralized to the bad ear
E. the preferred frequency of the tuning fork is 512 Hz

76. The following are useful in the management of inflammatory bowel disease (IBD) except:

A. sulfasalazine
B. prednisolone
C. dietary modification
D. antivirals such as aciclovir
E. antibiotics

77. What is the correct dose of epinephrine, when administered through an endotracheal tube?

A. 0.5 mg
B. 2.0 mg
C. 2–2.5 mg/kg
D. 0.1–1.5 mg/kg
E. 0.1 g

78. Which of the following symptoms are not consistent with irritable bowel syndrome (IBS):

A. abdominal pain
B. diarrhea
C. constipation
D. rectal bleeding
E. passage of mucus

79. The following are effective in the treatment of duodenal ulcers except:

A. *Helicobacter pylori* eradication
B. diet modification
C. ranitidine
D. omeprazole
E. steroids

80. The cognitive problems in Alzheimer disease are associated with a decrease in which of the following neurotransmitters:

A. serotonin
B. GABA
C. acetylcholine
D. glycine
E. substance P

81. All the following can be used to temporarily decrease intracranial pressure except:

A. intravenous mannitol
B. hypercapnia
C. hypocapnia
D. hypothermia
E. steroids

82. A 47-year-old complains of a 3-week history of lower abdominal pain. She denies any vaginal bleeding or discharge, and she describes no GI symptoms. She states that she found a site on the internet that stated that '25% of women will have fibroids over the course of their lives', and she is concerned that she therefore has a very high risk of having fibroids. The 25% figure that the patient read on the internet most likely represents:

A. the prevalence of fibroids
B. the incidence of fibroids
C. the sensitivity for fibroid detection
D. the true-positive rate of fibroid detection
E. none of the above

83. All of the following are causes of transudative pleural effusions except:

A. nephrotic syndrome
B. superior vena cava obstruction
C. myxedema
D. cirrhosis
E. pancreatic diseases

84. Which of the following statements about hypercalcemia is true:

A. the most common cause of hypercalcemia is malignancies
B. alkalinization of the urine favors nephrocalcinosis
C. EKG changes encountered in patients with hypercalcemia are: prolonged corrected QT and ST intervals, peaked T waves, arrhythmia and heart block
D. hypothyroidism can result in hypercalcemia due to increased bone resorption
E. thiazide diuretics are often necessary during volume repletion with saline to avoid pulmonary congestion

85. Target patients for pneumococcal vaccination are all of the following except:

A. patients 50 years old or older
B. patients on steroids or other immunosuppressive therapy
C. alcoholic patients
D. patients with diabetes mellitus
E. patients with chronic liver disease

86. You see a 60-year-old Caucasian woman in your office complaining of headaches, pain and stiffness in her shoulders, low grade temperature and weight loss. After completing her workup you make the diagnosis of polymyalgia rheumatica. Which of the following results is not consistent with your diagnosis:

A. erythrocyte sedimentation rate (ESR) of 105
B. normochromic normocytic anemia
C. negative rheumatoid factor
D. elevated creatinine phosphokinase
E. normal white cell count

87. The patient returns to your office 3 months later complaining of diffuse abdominal pain. On exam, her vital signs are stable but her abdominal exam reveals point tenderness in her left lower quadrant. On pelvic examination, her adnexa are non-palpable and you discuss the option of utilizing transvaginal ultrasound (TVU) to assess possible ovarian pathology. You find an abstract that suggests that, in cases where a woman has ovarian pathology, it can be detected 83% of the time by TVU. This figure best represents the:

A. specificity of TVU in detecting ovarian pathology
B. sensitivity of TVU in detecting ovarian pathology
C. positive predictive value of detecting ovarian pathology
D. negative predictive value of detecting ovarian pathology
E. none of the above

88. A 27-year-old woman comes to you after hearing a television news segment on the use of oral contraceptive pills. She tells you that the reporter quoted a study conducted by a local high school student that found that of a sample of 11 women taking OCPs, eight complained of headaches. She is concerned that her OCP use may lead to persistent headaches. The best approach to this concern is:

A. inform the patient that while you were unfamiliar with this study, it does sound as though OCPs cause headaches
B. tell the patient that this study was not sufficiently powered to detect the impact of OCPs on headaches
C. tell the patient that without a control group, the results of this study are of no value
D. discuss the differences between association and causality with the patient
E. tell the patient that while you would need to read the study in order to draw any conclusions, it appears that there are several flaws in both study methodology and reporting that should mitigate her concerns

89. A 42-year-old woman presents to your office on postoperative day 2 after a facelift with upper blepharoplasty. She complains of 'pressure' in her right cheek and difficulty speaking. You are concerned about the possibility of a hematoma and recall reading that the incidence of postoperative hematoma in facelift patients is approximately 5%, with a 95% confidence interval of 2.3–7.9%. Assuming that these numbers are correct, the 95% confidence interval means that:

A. 95% of patients will have a hematoma between 2.3% and 7.9% of the time
B. there is a 95% chance that this patient will have a hematoma between 2.3% and 7.9% of the time
C. the true value of the incidence of hematoma from this study lies within this range of values with a 95% degree of assurance
D. A and C
E. none of the above

90. You see a 51-year-old woman on postoperative day 3 after a left modified radical mastectomy with TRAM flap closure. She complains of breast tenderness and has drained

130 cc of bloody fluid from her Jackson Pratt drain over the past 24 hours. You are concerned about the potential amount of blood that this patient may be losing through her drain, and your attending physician asks you to find a study on the number of TRAM revisions that are performed in each hospital in the United States. When asked, the attending physician states that she wants only the mean and standard deviation from the study and does not need to see the remainder of the findings. The standard deviation is useful because:

A. it represents the amount of difference from the mean result that may be expected 90% of the time
B. approximately 95% of the probability mass falls within two standard deviations of the mean
C. it does not require a normal distribution to be meaningful
D. it may be interpreted independently of the mean
E. none of the above

91. You are interested in designing a study that will examine the incidence of complications after tumescent liposuction. You obtain records from 200 consecutive patients at a major teaching hospital and review them for any record of post-operative complications. This type of study is best described as a:

A. clinical trial
B. prospective study
C. retrospective study
D. non-randomized controlled trial
E. none of the above

92. You are reading a study on the incidence of mono-articular arthritis (MA), and you are interested in studying some of the risk factors that are associated with the development of MA. You find 160 patients with MA who were treated within your health system. You then select 180 patients with similar demographics who did not have MA and examine risk factors such as smoking, sexual activity, socioeconomic status and diet. This type of study is best described as a:

A. non-randomized controlled trial
B. retrospective clinical study
C. case-control study
D. crossover study
E. none of the above

93. The likely effect of a dopamine infusion at 5 μg/kg/min is:

A. peripheral vasoconstriction and marked tachycardia
B. systemic and renal vasoconstriction
C. dilation of renal blood vessels and marked peripheral vasoconstriction
D. increased cardiac output and a small increase in systemic vascular resistance
E. systemic vasodilatation and fall in blood pressure

94. You are interested in studying the role of antibiotic use in the treatment of chronic sinusitis. As part of a grant application, you propose to take the next 140 consecutive patients seen in your office who present with chronic sinusitis and assign them (using a lottery system) to either antibiotic or placebo, without knowing which patients are in each group. You then intend to follow the patients, who also do not know whether they are receiving placebo or antibiotic therapy, for 26 weeks and check for the number of recurrent episodes of sinusitis. This study is best described as:

A. prospective
B. randomized controlled trial
C. clinical trial
D. double-blind study
E. all of the above

95. Which of the following is true about the D-xylose absorption test:

A. it is a test that evaluates fat absorption
B. it is found abnormal in diseases affecting the mucosa of the small intestine
C. interpretation of the urinary values is more reliable than the blood level of the D-xylose
D. the test is not affected by diet or medications
E. all of the above are true

96. You are a member of the 'crash' team and are the first to arrive at the bedside. CPR has already been started by the nurses. You observe the rhythm shown (Figure 3). The rhythm shown is:

A. ventricular tachycardia
B. ventricular fibrillation
C. pulseless electrical activity
D. asystole
E. atrial fibrillation

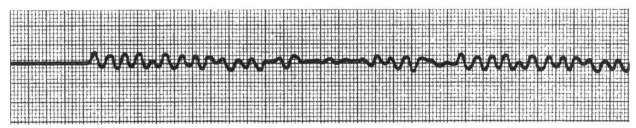

Figure 3 Refer to question 96

97. After stabilization the patient goes back into sinus rhythm briefly before going into the rhythm shown (Figure 4). What is the rhythm shown?

A. paced rhythm
B. idioventricular rhythm
C. nodal rhythm
D. slow atrial fibrillation

98. A 55-year-old man is seen in the ER for a broken arm. The rhythm strip is shown (Figure 5). What is the rhythm?

A. Wenckebach block
B. atrial fibrillation
C. atrial flutter
D. complete heart block
E. Mobitz 2:1 block

99. A 65-year-old male presents to his outpatient primary care physician with complaints of shortness of breath, and a history of 15 lb weight loss over the last 5 months as well as chronic low-grade fever. On posterior–anterior chest X-ray a moderate pleural effusion is noted on the left side. A thoracentesis is performed to diagnose the cause of the pleural effusion. Which of the following laboratory values is NOT considered a major criterion in differentiating exudative from transudative causes of pleural effusions?

A. pleural : serum protein > 0.5
B. pleural LDH > 200 U/l
C. pleural : serum LDH > 0.6
D. amylase > 300 U/l

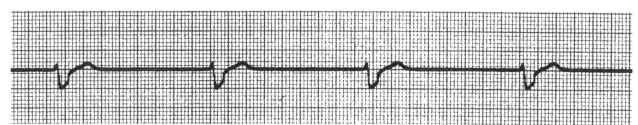

Figure 4 Refer to question 97

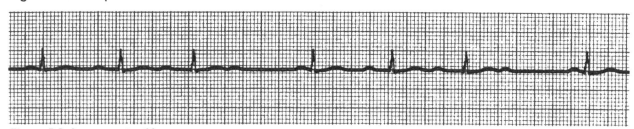

Figure 5 Refer to question 98

TEST TWO: ANSWERS

1. Answer: D

Although asthma itself can be life-threatening, that does not make pregnancy a contraindication. None of the medications that she is currently taking are considered teratogens.

Reference: Oski *et al.*, pp. 278–9, 782–6

2. Answer: B

Fat necrosis is usually found over a bony prominence and may be secondary to pressure or trauma during delivery. Most lesions resolve spontaneously, and require no intervention. Occasionally, a lesion may develop a calcification and require surgery.

Reference: Zitelli and Davis, p. 37

3. Answer: D

Three criteria should be met for the diagnosis of celiac sprue. These are 1) evidence of malabsorption; 2) an abnormal jejunal biopsy; and 3) clinical, biochemical and histologic improvement after a gluten-free diet. Approximately 90% of patients with untreated clinically symptomatic disease, and many patients with asymptomatic latent disease, have IgA and/or IgG antigliadin antibodies. Elevated antiendomysial antibodies are found in 90% of cases with active disease. Antireticulin antibodies are less sensitive but more specific. These antibodies are useful in following response to therapy, adherence to gluten-free diet and in screening of asymptomatic family members for the disease.

Reference: Fauci *et al.*, p. 1630

4. Answer: B

Crystals of monosodium urate are needle-shaped, negatively birefringent in polarized light and stand out brightly in a dark field. When a red plate compensator is used, the crystals are yellow when parallel to the axis and blue when perpendicular to the axis of the compensator. Calcium pyrophosphate dihydrate crystals are rhomboid and weakly positively birefringent. When a red plate compensator is used, the crystals are blue when parallel to the axis and yellow when perpendicular to the axis of the compensator.

Reference: Townes, p. 975

5. Answer: B

Lead poisoning is one of the most common and preventable pediatric health problems. The current recommendations, under the 1991 CDC guidelines, are for all children to have a screening of lead level at 2–3 years of age. The target organ systems include central nervous system, peripheral nervous system, kidney, bone marrow and erythroid cells. The constellation of lead poisoning includes gastrointestinal symptoms, coma, seizures, cerebral vasculitis, elevated intracranial pressure, microcytic hypochromic anemia, encephalopathy, renal dysfunction and motor weakness.

Reference: Zitelli and Davis, pp. 308–9; Oski *et al.*, pp. 842–6

6. Answer: A

Besides those listed in the question the key features include: brachydactyly, hypothyroidism, flat facial profile, small ears with small or absent ear lobes, speckling of the iris, upslanting of palpebral fissures, microcephaly and inner epicanthal folds. This is the most common autosomal chromosomal abnormality in liveborn infants. Frequency is estimated to be 1 in 700–1000 live births.

Reference: Zitelli and Davis, pp. 9–11; Oski *et al.*, pp. 2173, 2184

7. Answer: E

Horner syndrome can present as in this patient. A small pupil that does not dilate in dim illumination indicates involvement of the sympathetic nervous system. The diagnosis can be made with a cocaine test. A Horner pupil dilates less well than the normal pupil when both eyes have one drop of 10% cocaine instilled in them. A chest X-ray or CT of the chest is necessary to rule out a second-order neuron disorder due to a tumor such as thyroid adenoma, lung cancer, metastasis, etc. A third-order neuron disorder can occur secondary to an internal carotid dissection, given that this neuron travels along the carotid into the brain. Any previous surgery in the path of the sympathetic chain can disrupt or damage it as indicated. A cranial nerve palsy does not give an isolated lid droop and small pupil as in this patient. There are no restrictions in ocular motility with Horner syndrome.

Reference: Friedman *et al.*, pp. 203–4; Vander and Gault, pp. 209–11; Cullom and Chang, pp. 244–6

8. Answer: C

The onset and progression of puberty are variable. Tanner proposed a scale that describes the onset and progression of pubertal changes in boys and girls. Boys and girls are rated on a five-point scale. Boys are rated for genital development and pubic hair growth, and girls are rated for breast development and pubic hair growth.

Reference: Zitelli and Davis, pp. 280–2; Oski *et al.*, pp. 768–9

9.   Answer: E

The presence of a congenital aortic bicuspid valves causes aortic regurgitation and would cause a diastolic murmur. Systolic murmurs are caused by all the other mentioned conditions. Occasionally VSD can cause a diastolic murmur due to prolapse of an aortic cusp, resulting in progressive chronic aortic regurgitation.

Reference: Fauci *et al.*, pp. 199, 1320

10.   Answer: E

This patient probably has a metastasized bronchial carcinoid tumor. Bronchial adenomas are carcinoids in 80–90% of cases. They present as endobronchial lesions and are symptomatic for several years. Patients may have chronic cough, recurrent hemoptysis or obstruction with lobar collapse, pneumonitis or lung abscess formation. Bronchial carcinoids, like small cell lung cancers, derive from the APUD system (amine precursor and decarboxylation system). They may secrete hormones such as ACTH or vasopressin and cause paraneoplastic syndromes that resolve upon resection. Bronchial carcinoids can metastasize, usually to the liver, and may produce the carcinoid syndrome, with cutaneous flash, bronchoconstriction and diarrhea, and cardiac valvular lesions. Most of the tumors have a central endobronchial location and are visible by fiber-optic endoscopy. Because they are hypervascular, they can bleed profusely after bronchoscopic biopsy. Bronchial carcinoids require surgical removal because they can metastasize, be locally invasive, produce obstructive symptoms and produce a paraneoplastic syndrome. In the setting of a carcinoid syndrome urinary 5-hydroxy-indoleacetic acid levels are usually elevated. Vanillylmandelic acid is elevated in patients with pheochromocytoma.

Reference: Fauci *et al.*, pp. 561, 595

11.   Answer: A

Aerosolized pentamidine is not an acceptable treatment for PCP pneumonia. The pentamidine dose of 4 mg/kg/day has to be delivered by intravenous infusion. All the other regimens are acceptable treatments for PCP in a patient with sulfonamide allergies.

Reference: Gilbert *et al.*

12.   Answer: E

A marked and persistent fear of one or more social or performance situations, in which the person is exposed to unfamiliar people or to possible scrutiny by others and fears that he or she will act in a way that will be humiliating or embarrassing, is the essential feature of social phobia. Social phobia may be limited to a single specific stimulus (called the phobic stimulus), or may be generalized to almost all social situations. Common specific phobias include fear of public speaking, of eating or writing in public, or of using public lavatories.

Reference: DSM–IV, p. 416

13.   Answer: A

Migraine headaches are typically unilateral throbbing pain accompanied by nausea and vomiting. Visual disturbances including flashing (zigzag) lights, blurred vision, or a visual field defect that can last up to 20 minutes may precede a migraine and are referred to as a classic migraine (10% of cases). A positive family history is common including cyclic vomiting as a child. Migraine is more common in women and up to 70% of patients are female. Precipitating factors include any foods containing tyramine or phenylalanine (e.g. chocolate, wine), stress, birth control pills, bright lights, etc. Frequent severe headaches are treated prophylactically with amitriptyline, calcium channel blockers and propranolol.

Reference: Cullom and Chang, pp. 433–4; Friedman *et al.*, pp. 378–9

14.   Answer: A

Bilateral optic disc swelling may be due to increased intracranial pressure. A CT scan should be obtained to rule out an intracranial process such as tumor or mass. Once a mass is ruled out, a spinal tap should be done to rule out increased intracranial pressure. Swollen discs as a result of increased intracranial pressure are referred to as papilledema. Visual loss lasting seconds (transient visual obscurations), headache, double vision, nausea and vomiting may all occur. A decrease in visual acuity, usually mild in the acute setting, is rare. However, severe loss of vision can occur with chronic papilledema.

Reference: Kelley, p. 2356; Vander and Gault, pp. 223–4; Cullom and Chang, pp. 270–2

15.   Answer: D

Fluoroquinolones are contraindicated in children under 12 years of age as they interfere with cartilage and bony development at growth plates.

Reference: Oski *et al.*, p. 1219

16.   Answer: E

At this age the most probable cause of the pneumonia is *Staphylococcus aureus*, which colonizes and can become invasive within the first few weeks of life. By young childhood the primary infective organism is *Pseudomonas aeruginosa*. *Aspergillus* is a fungal infection that in adolescence usually colonizes the airways, causing allergic bronchopulmonary aspergillosis.

Reference: Zitelli and Davis, pp. 478–82; Oski *et al.*, pp. 1490–1

17. Answer: B

Teenage pregnancy is always difficult to manage, regardless of the established relationship a physician may have with the patient. It is important to make a timely diagnosis, provide medical information, and then either provide counseling or make a referral for counseling. Counseling should be unbiased and there should be a dialog directed at trying to involve the parents in an honest manner.

Reference: Oski et al., pp. 782–6

18. Answer: E

All of these findings are classic for 'shaken baby' syndrome. All of the findings have been found as part of other diagnoses, except for retinal hemorrhages. Although the uniqueness of this association has come under scrutiny recently, retinal hemorrhages have only occasionally been seen in children who have undergone cardiopulmonary resuscitation and had pre-existing malignant hypertension or coagulopathy.

Reference: Zitelli and Davis, pp. 144–6; Oski et al., p. 662

19. Answer: E

G6PD deficiency is an X-linked recessive disorder seen commonly in black men, characterized by episodic hemolysis in response to oxidant drugs (dapsone, primaquine, quinidine, quinine, sulfonamides and nitrofurantoin). The peripheral smear is minimally abnormal. The process is self-limited because the older red blood cells are removed and replaced with a population of young red blood cells with adequate functional levels of G6PD. Paroxysmal nocturnal hemoglobinuria is usually characterized by a decreased leukocyte alkaline phosphatase. Pyruvate kinase deficiency is a rare autosomal dominant recessive disorder that causes chronic hemolytic anemia, usually with onset in childhood. Splenomegaly and pigmented gallstones are present.

Reference: Tierney et al., pp. 475–6

20. Answer: B

The variability in symptoms throughout the day is the hallmark of myasthenia gravis. Edrophonium chloride, a short-acting anticholinesterase, causes improvement of the patient's symptoms with resolution of diplopia when administered intravenously. Myasthenia can mimic any nerve palsy. Once suspected, a chest MRI should be obtained to rule out a thymoma. In thyroid disease, there is no lid droop but lid retraction. Vitamin deficiency has no relevance to this diagnosis.

Reference: Vander and Gault, p. 216; Cullom and Chang, pp. 264–6

21. Answer: A

An isolated third nerve palsy and a dilated pupil in the presence or absence of a history of trauma is an emergency and one must rule out an aneurysm, particularly at the junction of the internal carotid and posterior communicating arteries. Emergent neurosurgical consultation should be obtained. If the neuroimaging studies (MRI/MRA) are negative, an angiogram should be obtained. A pupil sparing third nerve palsy is more likely to be vasculopathic, but patients with this condition also need to be followed very closely, initially, in the event of an evolving aneurysm. The differential diagnosis of a dilated pupil includes Adie's tonic pupil, pharmacologic, iris sphincter trauma, acute angle closure glaucoma and association with a third nerve palsy.

Reference: Wilson, pp. 136–8; Vander and Gault, pp. 212–13; Cullom and Chang, pp. 248–51

22. Answer: A

Males affected with fragile X syndrome are mentally retarded with borderline IQ. Physical features include long, wide protruding ears, long face, prominent jaw, flattened nasal bridge, a high arched palate, relative macrocephaly, hyperextensible joints, and macro-orchidism. Developmental problems include speech delay, short attention span, hyperactivity, and poor motor coordination. The fragile X gene is 80% penetrant in males and is 30% penetrant in females.

Reference: Zitelli and Davis, pp. 16–17

23. Answer: D

Testicular torsion is a true surgical emergency. There are two types – intravaginal or extravaginal – with the former being more common. Prompt surgical exploration and detorsion is mandatory as the testis may be irreversibly injured within 4 hours. Although additional investigations such as a technetium scan or ultrasound may be obtained, the delay in surgery is an unacceptable risk.

Reference: Zitelli and Davis, p. 520; Oski et al., p. 1766

24. Answer: A

The most likely diagnosis is ALS. He has cranial nerve involvement as well as both upper and lower motor neuron signs with fasciculations. These features, together with the patient's age and the chronicity of the clinical course, point towards ALS as the diagnosis. There is no sensory involvement. An EMG will help in the final diagnosis.

Reference: Samuels and Feske, pp. 474–9

25. Answer: A

Riluzole has been shown to delay the progression of ALS by 3 months. Trials are under way to assess the efficacy of this drug when given early in the disease. The other treatments mentioned have no effect in ALS. BDNF, a growth factor, has also recently been shown to have no effect on the progression of ALS.

Reference: Samuels and Feske, p. 478

26. Answer: A

The most likely diagnosis is MG. The history of blurred vision and axial weakness with ptosis and ophthalmoplegia support the diagnosis of MG. The diminishing reflexes are also typical of MG. There is also a chronic history of intermittent blurred vision suggesting intermittent ophthalmoplegia. Eaton–Lambert syndrome is a paraneoplastic disease and is characterized by distal weakness, increased strength and increasing reflexes on repetitive stimulation. This presentation does not support the diagnosis of ALS or depression.

Reference: Samuels and Feske, pp. 562–7

27. Answer: D

An MRI of the brain will be the least helpful in this patient as there is no evidence of a central nervous system problem. An EMG will show decrementing responses on repetitive stimulation. A CT of the thorax should be done to rule out a thymoma, which is present in 30% of myasthenics. Anticholinergic receptor antibodies are present in over 90% of patients and are a useful diagnostic tool.

Reference: Samuels and Feske, pp. 562–7

28. Answer: E

Aminoglycosides are contraindicated in MG as they can block neuromuscular transmission. Pyridostigmine is an acetylcholinesterase inhibitor and is useful in the long-term management of MG.

Reference: Samuels and Feske, pp. 562–7

29. Answer: A

Although the technology regarding the biochemistry and interpretation of tumor markers has evolved rapidly, their usefulness remains highly controversial. The use of CEA as a screening and prognostic indicator for colorectal carcinoma has been examined closely. It is unfortunately limited in its specificity, and it is elevated in a wide variety of conditions other than colorectal CA including hepatitis, cirrhosis, jaundice, COPD, pancreatitis, inflammatory bowel disease and renal failure. There are some reports linking smoking to increased CEA levels. The high level of false positives limits its usefulness as a screening tool. Several studies have established high levels of CEA as a prognostic indicator in patients undergoing surgical resection for colorectal carcinoma. A CT scan of the liver as part of a pre-operative evaluation is not indicated if liver enzyme and CEA levels are normal. After surgery is performed, the CEA level drops rapidly, and the first indication of recurrence is an elevated CEA level. There are reports of isolated falsely elevated CEA levels, so the test should be repeated if the result is deemed unusual or alarming. Many groups will use serially elevated CEA levels as a criterion for re-operation.

Reference: Sabiston, pp. 535–6

30. Answer: A

The likelihood of malignancy in this patient is exceedingly low. Solitary pulmonary nodules in non-smoking patients under the age of 35 are malignant in less than 1% of cases. Radiographic features can add weight to the presumptive diagnosis as well: 'popcorn' or 'bullseye' calcification patterns, consistent lack of growth, size under 1 cm, and a circumscribed appearance all lead toward a benign etiology. The low likelihood of malignancy does not warrant a tissue diagnosis; it would be remiss, however, to pass up the opportunity to review the progression of the lesion if a previous radiograph is available.

Reference: Fauci et al., pp. 558

31. Answer: D

Lung cancer is the most commonly occurring carcinoma in both men and women, and while SCC used to be the most common type, it now accounts for 30% of all lung cancers (adenocarcinoma accounts for 50% and small cell carcinoma for 15%). These cancers almost always originate in central lung fields, whereas adenocarcinomas more commonly occur peripherally or at the site of scarring. Smoking is by far the greatest risk factor for the development of SCC, and it is believed that other environmental risk factors (asbestos, radon, chromium, arsenic) act synergistically to increase the risk.

Reference: Greenfield, p. 1417

32. Answer: D

Increasing the sample size of a study is generally accepted to be the best method of increasing its power. Another method of increasing the power, that is not always possible to adjust, is increasing the proportion of participants with the event under study. For example, if one were studying MIs, it would be better (if possible) to study men aged 65–74 rather than women aged 30–40, since the incidence of MIs will clearly be higher in the former group. Matching controls does not have an effect on the power of a study.

Reference: Rosner, p. 215

33. Answer: D

CMV retinitis is the most common ocular infection, with an incidence of 20% per year noted in patients with CD4+ counts < 50 cells/μl. It is important to conduct a dilated fundus exam to evaluate for white patchy areas of necrosis, particularly along the vascular arcades with accompanying hemorrhages in the posterior pole. Prompt referral to an internist to co-ordinate systemic therapy to halt the progression of CMV retinitis with its associated complications – including retinal detachment and optic neuritis – is indicated. Therapy includes induction with high dose antiviral ganciclovir and foscarnet followed by maintenance therapy. The main side-effects include bone marrow suppression and renal toxicity, respectively. Cidofovir is another antiviral agent currently in use associated with nephrotoxicity. The mode of action is by inhibition of viral DNA polymerase. Recurrence is known to occur despite therapy since these agents are virostatic, not virucidal.

Reference: Vander and Gault, pp. 267–9; Friedman *et al.*, pp. 298–300; Cullom and Chang, pp. 391–2

34. Answer: A

A test should be both sensitive and specific. When testing for a virus such as HIV, the central concern is that one does not want to miss any cases of disease. Therefore, it is most important that a test be highly sensitive. A reasonably high false-positive rate (or low specificity), while undesirable, is far more palatable than compromising the sensitivity. It is also important to note that this is in reference to a screening test, rather than a diagnostic test. Diagnostic tests are often more specific than their screening counterparts.

Reference: Hennekens *et al.*, pp. 337–9

35. Answer: D

Herpes zoster ophthalmicus can be the first clinical manifestation of HIV, especially in a young individual. It represents a herpes zoster viral reactivation following initial childhood infection by chickenpox. Those with a negative history of chickenpox are at risk for infection. The virus lays dormant in the trigeminal ganglion. Vesicular lesions confined to one side of the face are a typical presentation. If the tip of the nose is involved, there is concern for ocular involvement since the nasociliary nerve innervates both these areas. An HIV test should be obtained. If positive, depending upon the patient's CD4 count, there is a risk for developing CMV retinitis, the most common opportunistic ocular infection in AIDS. In such a setting, appropriate antiviral therapy with either ganciclovir or foscarnet is in order.

Reference: Vander and Gault, pp. 69–70, 267–73; Cullom and Chang, pp. 81–4, 389–90

36. Answer: A

There are important clues in the history which suggest that an intracranial lesion needs to be excluded. His having been a lifelong smoker, with weight loss, change in behavior and seizure, points towards a metastatic brain lesion. Migraines, cluster headaches and tension headaches are not typically associated with the other features given in the question. An early morning headache, aggravated by straining, nausea and vomiting points towards raised intracranial pressure.

Reference: Samuels and Feske, pp. 1087–92

37. Answer: C

The first priority is to secure the airway. Once the airway has been secured then other assessment of the patient can begin. Breathing and circulation should be assessed next. Always remember ABC – airway, breathing, circulation.

Reference: Cummins, p. 1.5

38. Answer: E

Orbital cellulitis can present as noted in this patient. It is imperative to obtain a CT of the orbit and sinuses to rule out a subperiosteal abscess and sinus disease, or to rule out a foreign body. The patient should be admitted and started on broad spectrum antibiotics to cover both gram-positive and gram-negative, and anaerobic organisms and evaluated daily for improvement. If worsening is noted despite intravenous antibiotic coverage for at least 36 hours, a repeat CT scan of the orbit and brain should be obtained to look for an abscess, with prompt drainage if found. Indeed, in the presence of a stiff neck, a lumbar puncture should be obtained to rule out meningitis. Any diabetic patient that presents with a diagnosis of orbital cellulitis should be assessed for ketoacidosis. The nasal mucosa and palate should also be carefully evaluated for mucormycosis, a life-threatening infection of the orbit. Necrotic areas should be biopsied and the patient treated appropriately with amphotericin B.

Reference: Friedman *et al.*, pp. 12–14; Wilson, pp. 367–8; Cullom and Chang, p. 407

39. Answer: D

A rapid onset and progression of proptosis (globe displacement) in a healthy child requires urgent attention to rule out rhabdomyosarcoma, a malignant growth that arises from mesenchymal tissue and has the potential to metastasize. A CT scan will show bony orbital destruction. This child must be managed by an urgent biopsy. Mortality is 60% once the lesion extends to the orbital bones. Definitive treatment includes chemotherapy combined with local radiotherapy. Metastatic neuroblastoma occurs earlier in life and the child is usually systemically ill with a diagnosis of abdominal cancer. The location of the mass to the superior orbit makes this highly suggestive of rhabdomyosarcoma. Retinoblastoma may present with leukocoria or strabismus, but does not progress rapidly and usually does not present with proptosis. A teratoma usually presents at birth and with transillumination of the mass noted.

Reference: Friedman *et al*, pp. 16–17; Vander and Gault, pp. 237, 342–3; Cullom and Chang, pp. 162–5

40. Answer: E

In an orbital blowout fracture, the affected site is the orbital floor with sparing of the orbital rim. There is a risk of prolapse of the orbital contents into the maxillary sinus with entrapment. Symptoms include pain, local tenderness, double vision (that disappears when one eye is covered), and eyelid swelling after nose blowing. One can have loss of sensation in the distribution of the infraorbital nerve (ipsilateral cheek and upper lip), tenderness as well as nosebleed. The use of nasal decongestants can minimize this. Surgical repair is an issue only if there is persistent double vision in the primary or reading position after several days when tissue swelling has lessened or if a large fracture is present. Double vision upon presentation is not an indication for emergent surgical intervention.

Reference: Wilson, pp. 364–5; Friedman *et al.*, pp. 2–4; Cullom and Chang, pp. 38–9

41. Answer: C

In the setting of a ruptured globe, it is important not to manipulate the eye if there is evidence of penetration of the eye. Otherwise, there is a risk of extrusion of the eye contents by placing pressure on the globe. Make the patient n.p.o., cover the eye with a protective shield, ascertain the time of the last meal, and prepare for immediate surgical repair. MRI is contraindicated in the presence of an intraocular foreign body that may be metallic with risk of further destruction to the ocular tissues. A CT scan of the orbits and brain is indicated.

Reference: Wilson, pp. 359–60; Cullom and Chang, pp. 45–6

42. Answer: C

The convulsive episode appears unlikely to be an epileptic seizure, because of the forcible closing of the eyelids, the side-to-side movement of the head, the asynchronous and flailing movement of the arms and legs, and the ability of the patient to localize to pain during the spell. The lack of postictal confusion is also suggestive of non-epileptic events. There is also a history, going back several years, of many physical symptoms and complaints not adequately explained by a physical disorder or injury. The DSM–IV diagnosis of somatization disorder requires at least four pain symptoms: two gastrointestinal symptoms, one sexual/reproductive symptom and one pseudoneurologic symptom, all unexplained by medical conditions or injury. On the other hand, the essential feature of hypochondriasis is preoccupation with fears of having, or the idea that one has, a serious disease based on a misinterpretation of one or more bodily signs or symptoms. Factitious disorders are characterized by physical or psychological symptoms that are intentionally produced or feigned in order to assume the sick role. Factitious disorders are distinguished from malingering, in which the individual also produces symptoms intentionally but has a goal that is obviously recognizable when the environmental circumstances are known (e.g. the production of symptoms to avoid standing trial).

Reference. DSM–IV, pp. 442, 449, 471

43. Answer: E

The child has symptoms that may be consistent with juvenile rheumatoid arthritis with pauciarticular onset (fewer than five joints involved at initial diagnosis). Septic arthritis must be ruled out, especially when there is monoarticular involvement. An intensely red and tender joint, with systemic symptoms of fever, chills and malaise should prompt an arthrocentesis.

Reference: Zitelli and Davis, pp. 186–92

44. Answer: C

In making the diagnosis, the most important differentiation to make is periorbital (preseptal) cellulitis versus orbital (postseptal) cellulitis. The septum is a connective tissue reflection of periosteum that inserts into the eyelid and provides an anatomical barrier protecting the orbit. Any concern of orbital involvement, impairment of eye movement, or impairment of vision may mean an orbital cellulitis and should be immediately evaluated with a CT scan of the head. Any evidence of postseptal infection requires further evaluation by an ophthalmologist, blood cultures, intravenous antibiotics and often surgical intervention.

Reference: Zitelli and Davis, p. 712; Oski *et al.*, pp. 954–6

45. Answer: C

Besides providing appropriate medical care to the child, as the caregiver you must become the advocate for the child. This includes providing supportive social and psychological care for him/her. Such children are often confused and bewildered. Confrontation with parents or judgmental actions may further confuse the child and add to his/her general distrust.

Reference: Zitelli and Davis, pp. 133–75; Oski *et al.*, pp. 650–67

46. Answer: C

This patient most probably has thrombotic thrombocytopenic purpura characterized by the classic pentad: microangiopathic hemolytic anemia with fragmentation of erythrocytes and signs of intravascular hemolysis, thrombocytopenia, diffuse and nonfocal neurological signs, decreased renal function and fever. Patients have mild to severe anemia. The neurological and renal symptoms are usually seen with a low platelet count. Patients have proteinuria, fall in renal function and decline of urine output. Coagulation studies are normal as opposed to those in disseminated intravascular coagulation (DIC). TTP must be distinguished from ITP (idiopathic thrombocytopenic purpura) or Evans syndrome by the finding of fragmented red cells on smear and negative Coombs test.

Reference: Fauci *et al.*, pp. 668–9

47. Answer: C

Much research has been devoted to the optimal antibiotic for this common surgical problem. The mixed flora of the proximal colon usually prompts, perhaps not inappropriately, the use of broad-spectrum antibiotics to cover gram-positive, gram-negative and anaerobic flora. Cefazolin provides good coverage against gram-positive flora, but its coverage of gram-negative flora is inferior to that of higher generation cephalosporins. Ampicillin, gentamicin and metronidazole is an effective broad-spectrum regimen, but it has not shown any benefit over single-dose cefoxitin or cefotetan. Single-dose cefotetan has been shown to be as effective as three doses of cefoxitin with decreased cost of administration. It has broad coverage of gram-positive, gram-negative and anaerobic flora.

Reference: Sabiston, p. 966

48. Answer: C

Inguinal hernias are an exceedingly common surgical problem. They occur in 1–3% of all children, with a male:female predominance of approximately 6 : 1. Risk factors for the development of an inguinal hernia include prematurity, connective tissue disorder and a family history. The anatomical basis for the inguinal hernia is slightly different in the pediatric population – they are almost always the result of a failure of the processus vaginalis (the outpouching of peritoneum that coats the gubernaculum) to obliterate. This persistent channel allows for hernias or hydroceles to form at points along its path. Inguinal hernias in infants occur most commonly on the right side (56% vs. 27%) most probably because of the increased mass of developing visceral tissue (vena cava) located on the right side, which interferes with the descent of the right testicle. Unfortunately, inguinal hernias generally do not resolve without surgical intervention and the potential for incarceration and strangulation mandate early intervention. Delay is appropriate to secure appropriate facilities/expertise, or if the infant is significantly premature. The procedure involves ligation of the processus vaginalis superior to the internal inguinal ring; repair of the inguinal canal itself is not necessary. Recurrence is very rare, much less common than in the adult population.

Reference: Greenfield, pp. 2032–3

49. Answer: A

The natural healing course of primarily closed wounds includes a certain element of fibrosis and wound retraction. The best surgical technique for minimizing esthetic impact of the scar in this situation involves a modest amount of wound eversion to guard against the inevitable wound retraction. Wounds with a low infection risk can be closed primarily at any time up to 12–24 hours after they occur, while significantly contaminated wounds should be closed (after thorough irrigation) within 6 hours.

Reference: Singer et al.

50. Answer: B

The diagnosis of the acute abdomen is one of the true art forms of medicine, and there is no substitute for experience and intuition. That being said, there are certain principles that are based on review and analysis of large populations of patients. There are known risk factors, more important for discussion than diagnosis, and these include decreased water or dietary fiber intake, family history and recent infection. It is thought that the lymphoid tissue of the appendix becomes swollen in certain gastroenteritides, and this leads to luminal

obstruction. While there is an exception to every rule, essentially all patients with appendicitis will have anorexia and pain. Fever is usually absent, surprisingly enough. A non-operative approach is appropriate under certain circumstances. The presence of a distinct mass in the RLQ in the absence of systemic symptoms of fever or peritonitis implies a locally controlled infection. Such a peri-appendiceal abscess can be treated with observation and antibiotics or CT-guided drainage. Vigilant observation for progression of symptoms or signs of tachycardia is important.

Reference: Greenfield, p. 1254

51. Answer: A

Disseminated intravascular coagulation (DIC) is a complex and poorly understood phenomenon that occurs as a result of a disturbance of the blood's delicately balanced pro- and antithrombotic tendencies. Usually, a significant triggering mechanism is required to cause a DIC state – trauma, sepsis, and endotoxinemia are all commonly identified precipitants. Intravascular coagulation occurs as a result of any of a wide variety of stimulants; fibrinogen is cleaved by thrombin into fibrin (which becomes cross-linked into pairs) and fibrinopeptides A and B. This leads to falling fibrinogen levels, and an increase in FDPs, also known as fibrinogen split products (FSPs). As the process progresses, plasmin, usually held in check by plasmin activator inhibitor and α-2-antiplasmin, enzymatically degrades formed fibrin into several products including the d-dimer (a combination of the d segments from two cross-linked fibrin molecules). In severe DIC, plasmin degrades fibrinogen, releasing single d segments, as well as other fibrin products that have strongly anticoagulant properties. It is the fibrinogen level that most strongly correlates with the severity of bleeding.

Reference: Fauci et al., p. 740

52. Answer: D

Inguinal herniorrhaphy is the most commonly performed surgical procedure in this country, followed closely by cholecystectomy. Approximately 700 000 are performed each year, as a result of the fact that 25% of males and 2% of females will develop an inguinal hernia in their lifetime. The inguinal hernia is the most common hernia in both men and women, although the femoral hernia is more common in women than in men. Approximately 75% of all hernias are inguinal hernias, and of these the indirect inguinal hernia is twice as common.

Reference: Sabiston, p. 1219

53. Answer: D

The Child–Pugh classification of liver function defines the correlation between several parameters of ESLD and operative mortality. The classification into categories A, B and C is based on an aggregation of the following clinical and laboratory parameters: serum bilirubin, serum albumin, degree of ascites, degree of encephalopathy and nutrition. The serum transaminases are a poor indicator of hepatic function, and may be normal or even low in ESLD.

Reference: Kelley, p. 667

54.   Answer: B

Hypersensitivity reactions to local anesthetics are rare, and are more commonly associated with ester-type anesthetics (procaine, tetracaine – all those which have only one 'i' in the generic name) than with amide-type anesthetics (lidocaine, bupivicaine – all those which have more than one 'i' in the generic name). Sensitivity to one agent in the class usually generalizes to the entire class, but not to those in the other class. As long as you have confidence in the patient's history, it is acceptable to use a member of the non-offending class of local anesthetics.

Reference: Goodman, pp. 337–8

55.   Answer: A

This patient has classic signs of adrenal insufficiency. This problem is thought to occur in roughly 1 in 5000 inpatients – rare but not unknown. It may occur as a result of a wide variety of different causes including metastasis, tuberculosis, hemorrhage, amyloidosis or a previously subclinical primary (idiopathic) adrenal insufficiency. The diagnosis should be considered in patients who show cardinal signs of shock unresponsive to therapy, hyperthermia, hyponatremia with hyperkalemia, and abdominal pain/nausea. The diagnosis may be a zebra, but before letting a patient like this deteriorate for too long, an ACTH stimulation test should be administered. Dexamethasone is the corticosteroid of choice for patients in addisonian crisis. Dialysis should be considered in any patient with hyperkalemia, but this is not an intervention that addresses his primary problem.

Reference: Fauci *et al.*, pp. 2051–2

56.   Answer: A

The causal relationship between thymic tumors and MG is not fully elucidated, but the beneficial effect of thymectomy for patients developing this disorder is well established. Thymectomy is usually palliative as an adjunctive therapy for patients, especially young women with a short disease course. While thymoma and MG do not necessarily co-occur, the majority of patients (75%) with a thymoma either have or will develop MG within 10 years. The converse is not true – only 10–20% of patients with MG have a thymoma, although most have thymic hyperplasia, and a predisposition for the development of thymoma in the future. Thymomas are associated with paraneoplastic syndromes other than MG, including pure red cell aplasia, Cushing syndrome, and hypogammaglobulinemia, though these are much less common.

Reference: Greenfield, pp. 1469–70

57.   Answer: E

The mechanism of injury in this patient is typical for a traumatic aortic injury, and in spite of a set of vitals that are not alarming the index of suspicion for this problem should be high. There are 10 cardinal radiologic features suggestive of aortic injury on a chest X-ray, and these are widened mediastinum, apical pleural capping, pleural fluid, loss of aortic knob, NGT deviated to right, tracheal deviation, large hemopneumothorax, obliteration of space between PA and aorta, inferior displacement of left main bronchus, and elevation and right shift of right main bronchus.

If the radiograph confirms your suspicion, confirmation is needed, usually by a thoracic aortogram or transesophageal ultrasound. The decision of which modality to use should be directed by the resources most readily available owing to the emergent nature of this condition.

Reference: Gold, p. 180

58.   Answer: E

In a landmark review of the role of surgery for active endocarditis in 1982, Dinubile (as a medicine resident at the University of Pennsylvania) laid out the major and minor indications for operative intervention. These indications remain unchallenged and for the most part unmodified to this day. These major and minor criteria are listed below. Surgery is indicated for patients that satisfy a single major or three minor criteria:

Major	Minor
Progressive heart failure	CHF resolved with medical treatment
Significant failure	Single embolus
Multiple embolic episodes	Definite left-sided vegetations
Persistent bacteremia	Early mitral valve closure/flail valve
Fungal endocarditis	Early prosthetic endocarditis
Extravalvular foreign body	Nonstreptococcal
Development of heart block	GNR TV endocarditis
Purulent pericarditis	Persistent fever without cause
Valve dehiscence or obstruction	New murmur
Relapse	No good antibiotics available

Reference: Dinubile

59.   Answer: D

Because of the inevitably deleterious effects of aortic stenosis on myocardium, surgery should be considered for asymptomatic patients that meet certain criteria. The actual decision to operate is, of course, based on many factors other than the hemodynamic parameters yielded by the TEE. The parameters listed in items A–C are valid indications for an operative intervention, as is an aortic root diameter greater than 60 mm. It is possible in this patient that aortic stenosis has caused alterations in the structure of the heart that contribute to atrial fibrillation.

Reference: David

60. Answer: C

The SAG is considered by some gastroenterologists to be a better test than the total protein content of the ascitic fluid. The gradient correlates with portal hypertension. A gradient greater than 1.1 is characteristic of uncomplicated cirrhotic ascites; a gradient of less than 1.1 is seen in conditions associated with exudative ascites.

Reference: Fauci et al., pp. 255–7

61. Answer: A

Further workup of thin melanomas should be limited to a complete history and physical examination, as the risk of metastatic disease is very low. A baseline chest X-ray may be obtained. For patients with melanomas of 1 mm or thicker sentinel node mapping and biopsy should be considered and offered when available. Sentinel nodes can be identified in 80% of cases and histologic examination is 95% accurate in predicting involvement in the rest of the nodal basin. If metastatic disease is detected a full metastatic workup should be performed – CT scanning or MRI of the head and abdomen. If metastatic disease is not detected a chest radiograph should suffice. Recent studies have shown limited utility of chest radiography and blood work to detect recurrent disease at follow-up. The majority of recurrences were discovered by history and physical examination alone.

Reference: Baldor and Humphreys, pp. 27–37

62. Answer: B

The most serious adverse effect of tamoxifen is the increased incidence of endometrial cancer, similar to that in women receiving estrogen replacement therapy. This may be related to tamoxifen's estrogenic activity. The relative risk was 2.2 compared to the population-based rates of endometrial cancer. Most of the cancers were of low stage and grade, similar to those associated with estrogen therapy. The value of routine screening has not been established, but any woman with unusual bleeding should be promptly evaluated.

Reference: Osborne, pp. 1609–19

63. Answer: D

HCC is substantially less common in the US than in most other countries, largely owing to the lower incidence of hepatitis B virus infection. The most important etiologic factors are hepatitis B virus (HBV) infection (estimated 200–250 × risk), cirrhosis and exposure to toxins. HCV

infection has a link to HCC, but no correlation between HAV and HCC has been shown. While not useful as a screening test, AFP is elevated in 70–95% of patients with HCC. The diagnosis of hepatic malignancy is not a universal contraindication to transplantation; while the outcomes are worse than for most other indications, the procedure is still commonly performed.

Reference: Greenfield, pp. 583, 1015, 2135–8

64. Answer: D

Malrotation is a relatively common anomaly, and can present either acutely or incidentally. The findings are relatively characteristic – the intestinal viscera are found rotated in a clockwise (relative to the surgeon's view) direction. Ladd bands are thickened peritoneal attachments between the cecum and the posterior abdominal viscera that lie across and can restrict the second and third portions of the duodenum. Once these bands are divided, the intestinal contents should be un-rotated (in a counter-clockwise direction) to a natural (but not anatomic) position. The viscera will, of their own accord, assume a position that places the duodenum in the RLQ and the cecum in the LUQ. The malrotation repair should also fix the midgut down in these locations to prevent future rotation. Because of the extra-anatomic location of the cecum, the appendix is usually removed to avoid future diagnostic dilemmas.

Reference: Sabiston, pp. 1246–7; Greenfield, p. 2055

65. Answer: C

Five per cent dextrose solutions have 170 kcal/l. Maintenance intravenous fluids for a 70-kg patient should give 2.5 l of fluid per day, or 425 kcal. This amount of dextrose can stimulate sufficient insulin release to have a positive effect on protein synthesis.

Reference: Greenfield, p. 43

66. Answer: A

Causes of hypercalcemia include hyperparathyroidism, malignancy (due to a parathyroid-like hormone secreted by the neoplasm), thiazides, diuretic use and hyperthyroidism (thyroid hormone stimulates bone resorption) to name just a few. The characteristic findings of primary hyperthyroidism are commonly quoted in the maxim 'stones, bones, groans and psychiatric overtones'. There are, however, protean manifestations of hypercalcemia that include neurologic, gastrointestinal, cardiovascular and renal symptoms and signs. Hypertension is one of the less commonly noted clinical features, but is nevertheless frequently present. Hyperreflexia is seen in hypocalcemia, however, not in hypercalcemia (where you would see hyporeflexia). Remember Chvostek's and Trousseau's signs? These are commonly seen in post-thyroidectomy patients who may have suffered parathyroid gland injury or unintentional excision.

Reference: Greenfield, pp. 257–8

67. Answer: A

Primary hyperparathyroidism is most commonly (65%) a disease of a single parathyroid gland. Two glands are involved 15% of the time; three- and four-gland involvement each occur approximately 10% of the time.

Reference: Sabiston, pp. 659–60

68. Answer: A

The diagnosis is most probably Guillain–Barré syndrome, also known as acute inflammatory demyelinating polyneuropathy. The weakness and absence of reflexes following a febrile illness support the diagnosis. An elevated CSF protein without a pleocytosis and an EMG will help with the diagnosis.

Reference: Samuels and Feske, pp. 500–2

69. Answer: A

Plasmapheresis and intravenous immunoglobulins have been found to be efficacious in the treatment of GBS. For plasmapheresis-treated patients, the median time for ventilator support was reduced by 11 days and the time taken for unassisted ambulation was 2 months. Immunoglobulin treatmnt is as effective as plasmapheresis.

Reference: Samuels and Feske, p. 502

70. Answer: C

Verapamil is a calcium channel blocker and can cause profound hypotension. Intravenous calcium chloride can be used to treat this adverse effect. The other agents have not been shown to help in this case.

Reference: Cummins, 7.17

71. Answer: B

The vibrating tuning fork of preferred frequency 512 Hz is placed next to the pinna, and then placed on the mastoid bone when the patient can no longer hear. The patient is asked whether he can hear better when the fork is placed on the mastoid bone. If bone conduction is better or equal to air conduction then this is a negative Rinne's test, and this occurs in conductive hearing loss. In sensorineural hearing loss air conduction is better than bone, a positive Rinne's test. Note that mixed patterns can confuse the interpretation.

Reference: Bates, p. 211

72. Answer: E

The differential diagnosis of panic disorder (i.e. panic attacks not caused by a general medical condition or by a substance-related disorder) includes a variety of physical illnesses. A number of cardiac (e.g. arrythmias, angina pectoris), neurologic (e.g. partial complex seizures, vestibular dysfunction, diencephalic brain tumors), and endocrine (e.g. hyperthyroidism, hyperparathyroidism, pheochromocytoma) disorders are commonly associated with episodic symptoms that resemble panic attacks. Appropriate physical examinations or laboratory tests may help in establishing the correct etiology. Panic symptoms are commonly associated with intoxication with central nervous system stimulants (e.g. caffeine, cocaine, amphetamines), or with cannabis, as well as with withdrawal from central nervous system depressants (e.g. barbiturates, benzodiazepines, alcohol). However, if the panic attacks continue to occur outside the context of the substance intoxication or withdrawal, a diagnosis of panic disorder should be considered. Epidemiological associations have been noted between panic attacks and irritable bowel syndrome, COPD and mitral valve prolapse, but the etiologic relationship between any of these entities remains unclear. No association between panic attacks and shift in sleep phase has been described.

Reference: DSM–IV, pp. 400–2, 436–41; Winokur and Clayton, pp. 142–3

73. Answer: D

Cataplexy is a temporary paralysis of the somatic musculature (sudden loss of muscle tone) during bouts of laughter, anger and other strong emotional states. Some attacks of cataplexy are partial, e.g. involving only the jaw muscles, but they can involve the neck (causing the head to fall), or legs (causing the knees to buckle or the patient to fall to the ground), and they always occur with perfect preservation of consciousness. The attacks are brief, lasting seconds or a minute or two, but on rare occasions the atonia can last several hours (status cataplexicus). This syndrome is pathognomonic of narcolepsy, a disease characterized by daytime sleepiness, sleep attacks, sleep paralysis, cataplexy, and hypnopompic and hypnagogic hallucinations. Narcolepsy is caused by a disturbance in the architecture of sleep such that REM periods occur in the absence of the preceding slow sleep stages. Although the genes and mode of inheritance are not identified, a genetic predisposition has been established in association with the HLA-DR2 antigen, which is present in almost 99% of patients with the full clinical syndrome. Cataplexy needs to be distinguished from drop attacks and atonic seizures, both manifestations of epilepsy, in which consciousness is abolished temporarily. Periodic paralysis is an inherited derangement of potassium metabolism resulting in episodic hypokalemia, which is associated with slow development, over the course of hours, of trunk and limb weakness which can result in total paralysis, but which also subsides completely over the course of hours or days. Catatonia is a clinical syndrome, usually part of schizophrenia or bipolar disorder, characterized by motoric immobility (as evidenced by catalepsy or stupor) or excessive motor activity (that appears purposeless and not influenced by external stimuli), extreme negativism (an apparently motiveless resistance to all instructions, or maintenance of a rigid posture against attempts to be moved), mutism, peculiarities of voluntary movement (stereotyped movements, posturing, mannerisms or grimacing) and echolalia or echopraxia. The essential feature of dissociative states is a disruption in the usually integrated functions of consciousness, memory, identity or perception of the environment. The disturbance may be sudden or gradual, transient or chronic, and the categories include amnesia, fugue, identity and depersonalization disorders.

Reference: DSM–IV, pp. 288–9, 477; Adams *et al.*, pp. 314–17, 1161

74. Answer: A

Chronic use of aminoglycosides can cause sensorineural damage. Wax, otosclerosis or a perforated immobilized ear drum can cause conduction loss. The commonest cause is wax.

Reference: Bates, p. 211

75. Answer: D

A tuning fork of preferred frequency 512 Hz is placed on the vertex of the skull and the patient is asked to identify the ear that the vibration is best heard in. In conduction loss, sound lateralizes to the impaired ear. Because the ear is not distracted by room noise, it can detect vibrations better than normal. In sensorineural loss, sound lateralizes to the good ear. The impaired inner ear is less able to transmit impulses no matter how the noise is transmitted to it. Mixed loss can make interpretation difficult.

Reference: Bates, p. 178

76. Answer: D

Antivirals have no proven role in the management of ulcerative colitis. However antibiotics such as metronidazole and ciprofloxacin are used in the treatment of inflammatory bowel disease. Sulfasalazine and other 5-aminosalicylates, steroids and dietary modification are all useful in the management of IBD.

Reference: Kelley, pp. 742–3

77. Answer: B

The intravenous dose is 1 mg. In general twice the intravenous dose of epinephrine should be used if given by endotracheal route.

Reference: Cummins, p. 2.3

78. Answer: D

Rectal bleeding, fever and weight loss are not clinical features of irritable bowel syndrome and should alert the clinician to consider other underlying disorders. However, diarrhea, constipation, abdominal pain and bloating, passage of mucus and alteration in stool frequency and consistency are all symptomatic criteria for IBS. There are no pathognomonic features of IBS and the clinician has to rely on recognition of positive features and exclusion of other disorders.

Reference: Kelley, pp. 708–9

79. Answer: E

Steroids may exacerbate duodenal ulcers and care must be taken when using steroids in patients with a history of duodenal ulcers. Dietary modification, proton inhibitors and the H_2 antagonists are all useful in management. *Helicobacter pylori* eradication is the most effective means for preventing ulcer recurrence.

Reference: Kelley, pp. 697–8

80. Answer: C

There is a decrease in the amount of acetylcholine in the brains of patients with Alzheimer disease. The nucleus of Meynert and the pathways from this nucleus are particularly affected. Glycine is an important cofactor at NMDA receptors and is an important inhibitory transmitter in the spinal cord. Serotonin is involved in many pathways and appears to be important in depression. Substance P plays a role in pain. GABA is an important inhibitory neurotransmitter in the brain.

Reference: Bradley *et al.*, p. 879

81. Answer: B

The osmotic diuretic mannitol is a useful agent in the management of raised intracranial pressure and works by decreasing intracranial volume by reducing brain water. Hypothermia, hypocapnia and pentobarbitol coma are also employed for this purpose. Hypercapnia causes vasodilatation and may therefore increase intracranial pressure. Corticosteroids reduce edema around intracranial tumors.

Reference: Samuels and Feske, p. 821

82. Answer: B

The prevalence of a disease provides a reference for the number of people with a disease at a given moment in time. It therefore provides an estimate that may be used to assess the probability (i.e. risk) that someone will have a disease at a given point in time. Its formula is given by P = number of existing cases/total population at a given point in time. Incidence, however, quantifies the number of new cases that occur over a specified time period. Its formula is given by I = number of new cases in a given period of time/total population at risk of acquiring the disease. Therefore, an important distinction between these two measures is that incidence reflects the number of incident cases over a given time period while prevalence reflects a snapshot that reveals something of the impact of a disease at a given point in time. Secondly, incidence, by definition, has in the denominator only those members of a population at risk of acquiring the disease or condition, while prevalence includes the entire population in the denominator. Sensitivity and true-positive rates are measures of the efficacy of a test rather than measures of disease frequency, and therefore clearly are not possible answers to this question. Because the 25% figure reflects the percentage of women who will acquire a disease over a specific time period, it represents the (cumulative) incidence of acquiring leiomyomata.

Reference: Hennekens *et al.*, pp. 64–6

83. Answer: E

Common causes of transudative effusions are: congestive heart failure, cirrhosis, nephrotic syndrome, peritoneal dialysis, superior vena cava syndrome, myxedema and pulmonary emboli. Pancreatic diseases are a cause of exudative pleural effusions.

Reference: Fauci *et al.*, p. 1475

84. Answer: B

The most common cause of hypercalcemia is hyperparathyroidism. Malignancies (squamous cell lung cancer, breast cancer, renal cell cancer) are the second most frequent cause of hypercalcemia. Hyperthyroidism can cause hypercalcemia by stimulating osteoclastic bone resorption. Alkaline urine decreases the solubility of calcium phosphate complexes and favors nephrocalcinosis. EKG changes encountered in hypercalcemia are shortened QT intervals, broader T waves, and first degree AV block. Thiazide diuretics decrease calcium excretion and can cause hypercalcemia. Treatment of hypercalcemia consists of fluid repletion, use of furosemide (a diuretic that is calciuretic) and administration of biphosphonates or calcitonin.

Reference: Greenberg *et al.*, p. 110

85. Answer: A

Target patients for pneumococcal vaccination are patients 65 years old or older, who are living in the community or in a skilled nursing facility or nursing home, patients who are taking steroids or other immunosuppressive therapy or chemotherapy, patients who are HIV-positive or have AIDS, alcoholics and post-transplant patients. The vaccination is recommended in patients who have chronic cardiovascular or pulmonary disorders, splenic dysfunction or asplenia, chronic renal failure, nephrotic syndrome, diabetes mellitus, chronic liver disease, hematologic malignancies, metastatic malignancies or congenital immunodeficiencies.

Reference: Tierney *et al.*, p. 1170

86. Answer: D

Polymyalgia rheumatica is a clinical diagnosis based on pain and stiffness of the shoulder and pelvic girdle area, frequently associated with fever and weight loss. Polymyalgia

rheumatica and giant cell arthritis frequently coexist. Anemia and elevated ESR are almost always present. In contrast to polymyositis, polymyalgia does not cause muscle weakness or a rise in muscle enzymes. In older patients with fever of unknown origin, an elevated ESR and a normal white cell count, giant cell arthritis must be considered even in the absence of specific features such as headache and jaw claudication.

Reference: Rudy and Kurowski, pp. 433, 466

87. Answer: B

Sensitivity and specificity are both measures of the validity of a screening test. Sensitivity is the probability of a positive test result if the disease is truly present. Specificity is the probability of screening negative if the disease is truly absent. A highly specific test will result in a relatively low number of false-negative results. The positive and negative predictive values assess whether or not an individual actually has the disease given the results of a screening test. The predictive values therefore are measures of the feasibility of a screening test rather than of the validity of the screening test results. When assessing the implications of a given result on an individual patient, the sensitivity and specificity should be considered; when evaluating a screening test as a screening test (i.e. whether the test should be adopted for widespread use), the positive and negative predictive values should be considered. In this case, the 83% reflects the sensitivity of the test since it is the probability of detecting the disease given that disease is actually present.

Reference: Schoenfeld *et al.*; Hennekens *et al.*, pp. 332–5

88. Answer: E

Even if an association between headaches and OCP use could be demonstrated without a doubt, concluding a causal relationship between the two would not necessarily follow directly. Causality cannot be conclusively determined from this study, and while there are several features of a relationship that suggest causality – such as biological plausibility, presence of a dose–response relationship, and temporal association between two factors – none of these is sufficient to prove causality. Statistical power relates to both the sample size and the frequency of the study endpoint (e.g. is it rare?). A control group would be helpful here, but studies may demonstrate mildly compelling results even without a control group (i.e. clearly headache should not be present in every patient). In this case, a study conducted by a high school student would probably not have adhered to any standard epidemiological principles. A sample size of 11 is most probably inadequate, although there are situations where such small sample sizes may provide sufficient power to represent an effective study (e.g. in cases where a very large difference between the two groups under study is expected).

References: Hennekens *et al.*, pp. 3–15

89. Answer: C

Confidence intervals are often utilized in lieu of *p* values for several reasons. Because *p* values are very sensitive to the sample size, relatively small differences may have low *p* values if the sample size is sufficient whereas even large differences, in the context of a small sample size, may have high *p* values. Confidence intervals are preferred by many epidemiologists because they adequately demonstrate the role of sample size; the wider the confidence interval, the smaller the sample size. Therefore, an unimpressive result with a wide confidence interval may actually be promising whereas an unimpressive result with a narrow confidence interval suggests that there is little if any effect and that the perceived difference may be largely due to the large sample size. The confidence interval represents the range of values within which the true value lies with a 95% degree of assurance. It does not, however, mean that 95% of patients will experience an event between *x* and *y*% of the time.

Reference: Hennekens *et al.*, pp. 252–3

90. Answer: B

The standard deviation, or the square root of the variance, provides a measure of the spread of a variable around the mean. It therefore is predicated on having a normal (or approximately normal) distribution and of course is relevant in the context of its relationship to the mean value. From a clinical standpoint, it is useful because approximately 68% of the probability mass will fall within one standard deviation of the mean, and approximately 95% will fall within two standard deviations of the mean.

Reference: Rosner, pp. 163–4

91. Answer: C

'Clinical trial' is a generic term usually referring to a randomized controlled trial. The terms prospective and retrospective are used to denote the temporal relationship between when the study was initiated and when the data were collected. Because the study under discussion here was conducted on events that occurred before it was initiated, it is best considered a retrospective study. There is clearly no control group or randomization in this study.

Reference: Hennekens *et al.*, pp. 178–212

92. Answer: C

A non-randomized controlled trial would, by definition, be prospective. While this study is retrospective, it would better be described as a case-control study. Patients are selected by whether or not they have experienced the event (MA). The presence of previous exposure is subsequently assessed and differences in exposure between the event-positive and event-negative groups are examined. A crossover study does not, by definition, involve the use of a control group.

Reference: Hennekens *et al.*, pp. 178–212

93. Answer: D

Dopamine has β-1 and α effects. The effect of dopamine depends on the dose. A dose of 1–2 μg/kg/min of dopamine has a direct effect on dopaminergic receptors to produce cerebral, renal and mesenteric vasodilatation, and urine output may increase. At doses between 2 and 10 μg/kg/min the β-1 effect causes an increase in cardiac output and partly antagonizes the α effect of vasconstriction on the peripheral vasculature. At higher doses there is a marked increase in renal mesenteric peripheral arterial and venous vaso-constriction.

Reference: Cummins, p. 8.3

94. Answer: E

This study is prospective, it is randomized and controlled, and it is double-blind. If forced to choose from amongst these options, the best answer would be B, because it best describes the study. Still, because all of these descriptors are actually correct, answering all of the above is the best choice.

Reference: Hennekens *et al.*, pp. 178–212

95. Answer: B

The D-xylose absorption test is a test used to evaluate carbohydrate absorption. The patient has to ingest 25 g of D-xylose and this is followed by measurement of the D-xylose levels on a 5-h urine collection – a level of 26 mmol/l (4.0 g/l) or greater is considered to be normal. Low levels may be obtained in patients with ascites, intestinal bacterial overgrowth, or renal insufficiency, after administration of certain drugs and most commonly when urine collection is incomplete. To prevent difficulties in interpreting the test it is advisable to determine the blood xylose level 2 h after ingestion of xylose. A blood level of 2 mmol/l or greater indicates normal absorption of D-xylose. Abnormal absorption is most commonly found in disorders affecting the mucosa of the proximal small intestine, such as celiac sprue and tropical sprue.

Reference: Fauci *et al.*, p.1614

96. Answer: B

The rhythm shows ventricular fibrillation. Immediate unsynchronized DC cardioversion at 200 J is required.

Reference: Cummins, pp. 1.17, 4.6

97. Answer: B

The rhythm shown is idioventricular rhythm. The electrical activity originates from the ventricles. Rates greater than 75 beats per minute are called accelerated idioventricular rhythm.

Reference: Hampton, pp. 86, 283

98. Answer: A

The rhythm shown is Wenckebach block. The P–R interval gets progressively longer and is then followed by a non-conducted P wave. This rhythm is of physiological interest and is not thought to be clinically important.

Reference: Hampton, p. 100

99. Answer: D

Light's definitive work in differentiating exudative from transudative pleural effusion has yielded a set of diagnostic criteria which has important clinical ramifications. The criteria that bear his name include items A–C in the question but not item D. The differentiation is not merely an exercise; 83% of transudates are hydrostatic in origin (usually CHF) while 43% of exudates are malignant.

Reference: Light, pp. 129–53

TEST THREE

Satellite health center

1. A 4-year-old is brought to your clinic. The parents are concerned that the child does not function at the level of other 4-year-olds and is hyperactive. Your physical examination is strongly suggests features consistent with fetal alcohol syndrome. These features include all of the following except:

A. well defined philtrum
B. thin, smooth upper lip
C. prominent ears
D. microcephaly
E. short palpebral fissures

2. During a health maintenance physical examination you perform a developmental assessment. The child can stand alone and take two steps, hold a crayon and scribble, stack two blocks, and speaks a number of words with an occasional two-word sentence. The appropriate age of this child is:

A. 6 months
B. 12 months
C. 18 months
D. 24 months
E. 30 months

3. All of the following are risk factors for development of breast cancer except:

A. family history
B. early menarche
C. late menopause
D. alcohol consumption
E. multiparity

4. A 13-year-old boy is seen at your office for a thyroid nodule noticed incidentally on a routine physical exam by his pediatrician. On exam, his thyroid is felt to have a 1.5×1.5 cm nodule in the right lobe of his thyroid, and a background of multinodular tissue. An ultrasonograph confirms these findings. He has one maternal aunt with a known medical history of papillary thyroid CA (unknown variant),

but no known exposure to any significant radiation. Which of the following factors do NOT increase the likelihood that his thyroid nodule is malignant:

A. his age
B. the presence of background multinodularity
C. positive family history
D. all of the above increase the likelihood that the nodule is malignant

5. What is the most appropriate next test to differentiate between a benign and a malignant thyroid nodule?

A. radioactive thyroid scan
B. fine needle aspiration
C. excisional biopsy
D. thyroid stimulating hormone (TSH) level

6. A 9-year-old is seen in your clinic with the complaint of facial pain over his maxilla bilaterally. Over the past month he has had a cough that is more pronounced when he is trying to sleep. Upon physical examination there is tenderness with percussion over the maxillary regions, and inspection of the nares reveals a glistening mucosal pedunculated growth. In addition to a CT scan of the nasopharynx for evaluation of sinusitis, the second diagnostic test to order is:

A. radiographs of sinuses
B. chest radiograph
C. nasal swab for Gram stain and culture
D. sputum specimen for Gram stain and culture
E. sweat chloride

7. A 14-year-old comes to your clinic. His mother complains that his school performance has declined recently and that he has started soiling his underwear. In talking with the boy he relates that his parents are always arguing and he is worried they will divorce. He is embarrassed about his fecal incontinence, occasionally has intermittent periumbilical pain, but otherwise feels good. On examination, his height and weight are at the 75th percentile for age, abdomen is soft, nontender, with stool palpable in the LLQ, and normal anal sphincter tone. Otherwise, his examination, including neurologic, is normal. Your initial evaluation includes a barium enema that reveals a large dilated colon, including

dilation of the rectum to the anal verge. Blood tests show a normal white blood cell count and normal erythrocyte sedimentation rate. Your presumptive diagnosis is:

A. Hirschsprung disease
B. encopresis
C. anterior displacement of the anus
D. spina bifida occulta
E. inflammatory bowel disease

8.   All live viral vaccinations are contraindicated in patients with the following entities except:

A. common variable immunodeficiency (CVID)
B. severe combined immunodeficiency (SCID)
C. HIV
D. currently receiving chemotherapy
E. X-linked agammaglobulinemia

9.   A student from the local university comes to the clinic for a carbamazepine level. The following are known side-effects of carbamazepine except:

A. rash
B. neutropenia
C. diplopia
D. gum hyperplasia

10.   During a routine school physical, you notice decreased femoral pulses in a 12-year-old child. Upon obtaining four extremity blood pressures you find that the upper extremities are hypertensive with decreased blood pressures in the lower extremities. The physical examination is otherwise unremarkable. The child relates a normal activity level and is in fact one of the top athletes in his grade. Your next management step is:

A. chest radiograph
B. referral to a pediatric cardiologist
C. obtain blood tests and urinalysis
D. initiate antihypertensive medications
E. dietary control of hypertension

11.   The following statements about antimicrobials are all true except:

A. tetracycline can be deposited in growing bones
B. gentamicin can cause hearing loss
C. nitrofurantoin can cause peripheral neuropathy
D. metronidazole can cause peripheral neuropathy
E. the combination of amoxicillin and clavulanic acid is not clinically useful

Office

12.   A 20-year-old white woman presents to your office with a moderately red eye, and a meiotic pupil on the right side. She has had these symptoms for 2 weeks. The patient acknowledges mild pain and photophobia but denies any history of seasonal allergies or recent upper respiratory tract infection. You further elicit a history of arthritis. There is no evidence of an afferent pupillary defect or discharge noted with minimal tearing. The most likely diagnosis is:

A. acute glaucoma
B. bacterial conjunctivitis
C. allergic conjunctivitis
D. viral conjunctivitis
E. uveitis

13.   A patient on chronic steroid inhalers and p.o. steroids is at risk for all of the following except:

A. formation of cataracts
B. exacerbation of a herpes corneal infection
C. elevation of intraocular pressure
D. slow healing of a corneal abrasion
E. optic neuritis

14.   A 65-year-old patient presents to your clinic complaining of several episodes of visual loss in the right eye – lasting about 20 minutes with full recovery – over the last few days. In your evaluation, you should:

A. evaluate the fundus for evidence of retinal emboli
B. obtain an electrocardiogram and echocardiogram
C. schedule a carotid Doppler test
D. check blood pressure in both sitting and standing position
E. all of the above

15.   A 24-year-old female presents to your office with a complaint of being unable to see to the sides. You determine upon confrontation field testing complete loss of visual field in the right half of the right eye and left half of the left eye. The lesion most likely:

A. involves the optic tract
B. is localized to the temporal lobe
C. is a manifestation of a pituitary adenoma
D. is a manifestation of a craniopharyngioma
E. is a classic presentation of hysteria

16.   A 40-year-old patient presents with an inability to see superiorly to the left. Upon confrontation you determine a bilateral left-sided superior visual field defect. You determine the presence of formed hallucinations. The site of lesion is most probably located in the:

A. occipital lobe
B. chiasm
C. optic tract
D. temporal lobe
E. parietal lobe

17. A 60-year-old coal miner presents with a complaint of episodes of bronchospasm and decreased libido. You determine he has recently gone onto a disability benefit owing to a chronic back problem and has been newly diagnosed with hypertension and glaucoma for which he has been prescribed an oral calcium channel blocker and a topical β–blocker eye drop once a day. The most appropriate step would be to:

A. obtain a psychiatric consultation for possible anxiety disorder due to new precipitating stress factors in his life
B. consider therapy with sildenafil after a complete medical examination
C. discontinue the heart medication
D. place the patient on a bronchodilator inhalant to treat episodes of bronchospasm
E. discontinue the eye drops

18. A 42-year-old housewife presents to your office. She voices concern of redness in her right eye upon awakening. You determine normal visual acuity and pupil exam, with no associated eye pain or discharge. You should:

A. reassure the patient that this will resolve over time and prescribe artificial tears
B. inquire if the patient has a history of seasonal allergies
C. determine if the patient is on warfarin
D. all of the above
E. none of the above

19. Which of the following statements regarding endotracheal intubation are incorrect?

A. it decreases the risk of aspiration
B. it should be performed before defibrillation for the patient in VF
C. it provides a route for administration of some medications
D. it should not be attempted by inexperienced professionals

20. A 55-year-old woman presents to your office with complaint of loss of appetite, tingling in the fingers and feeling depressed. The patient reports using a number of medications for glaucoma management. The most likely candidate is:

A. timolol (β-blocker)
B. brimonidine (α-2-agonist)
C. acetazolamide (carbonic anhydrase inhibitor (CAI))
D. latanoprost (prostaglandin)
E. the patient may be having menopause and requires estrogen replacement therapy

21. A patient presents to your office with unevenly sized pupils. All of the following may be associated with this except:

A. Horner syndrome
B. Adie's pupil
C. physiologic
D. trauma
E. relative afferent pupillary defect (RAPD)

22. A 4-month-old infant is brought to your office because the mother is concerned about the infant's emesis with feeding and states the child is not gaining weight. The child is fed regular whey and casein protein-based formula. On physical examination the child is well developed and at the 50th percentile for height, weight and head circumference. The most appropriate action is:

A. reassurance and support that this is normal, change formula to another brand
B. reassurance and support that this is normal, no change in formula
C. reassurance and support that this is normal, change to a soy protein-based formula
D. reassurance and support that this is normal, change to a lactose-free formula
E. reassurance and support that this is normal, change to an elemental formula

23. A 16-year-old girl comes to your office complaining of acne. She has been on topical antibiotics for 3 months with minimal improvement. On examination the teenager has a number of comedones, and pustules on her cheeks and forehead. On her right cheek she has two deep cystic papules that are firm and tender to the touch. The next step in management is:

A. systemic oral antibiotics
B. benzoyl peroxide topical therapy
C. retinoic acid topical therapy
D. referral to a dermatologist
E. continue current management and re-evaluate in 2 weeks

24–26. A 6-month-old baby is admitted to the hospital following poor weight gain and repeated chest infections. Cystic fibrosis is suspected.

24. Which of the following results of the sweat test would fit with the diagnosis of cystic fibrosis:

A. low sodium and normal chloride
B. high sodium and high chloride
C. low sodium and high chloride
D. high sodium and normal chloride

25. Features of cystic fibrosis include all of the following except:

A. meconium ileus
B. pancreatic failure
C. bronchiectasis
D. diabetes
E. hypothyroidism

26. Which statement is correct regarding the inheritance of cystic fibrosis?

A. autosomal recessive, so one in six offspring of carrier parents will be affected
B. autosomal dominant, so one in two offspring of carrier parents will be affected
C. autosomal recessive, so one in four offspring of carrier parents will be affected
D. is X-linked
E. severity of the disease is virtually constant and does not vary much between individuals

27. Symptoms identical to a manic episode can be caused by:

A. corticosteroids
B. electroconvulsive therapy
C. tricyclic antidepressants
D. light therapy
E. all of the above

28. Melancholic features of major depression include all the following except:

A. loss of pleasure in almost all activities
B. early morning awakening
C. marked psychomotor retardation
D. leaden paralysis

29. In a patient with major depression, features that predict a better response to MAOIs include:

A. the patient's mood brightens in response to positive events
B. prominent somatic anxiety
C. increased appetite and weight gain
D. leaden paralysis (i.e. heavy, leaden feeling in limbs)
E. all of the above

30. Binge eating is associated with:

A. Kleine–Levin syndrome
B. anorexia nervosa
C. bilateral mesial temporal lobe lesions
D. bulimia nervosa
E. B and D

31. A 5-day-old is brought to your office, as the mother is concerned about a bruise on the face. The birth history reveals that the birth was a vaginal delivery with the assistance of forceps. Physical examination reveals a well-circumscribed, firm nodule the size of a nickel with purplish discoloration on the right cheek. The most appropriate next step is to:

A. refer to a plastic surgeon
B. offer reassurance to the mother that this is normal and will resolve spontaneously
C. obtain a skull radiograph
D. refer them to a geneticist for screening and counseling
E. obtain a biopsy

32. A 2-year-old boy is brought to your office, with a mother complaining of a diaper rash. Initially, you notice the child sitting restlessly and pulling at his diaper trying to scratch his buttocks. Physical examination is only remarkable for an erythematous and inflamed perianal region. The diagnostic test of choice is:

A. stool for leukocytes
B. stool for ova and parasites
C. stool culture
D. perianal tape test
E. gastric string test

33. Parental and child risk factors for child abuse and neglect include all of the following except:

A. child's age over 3 years
B. parental history of being an abused child
C. infants separated from their mothers at birth because of illness or prematurity
D. children seen as difficult or different
E. parents with poor socialization and lack of trust in others

34. A newborn is brought to your office for a 1-week check-up. He is a breast-fed infant and is noticeably jaundiced; otherwise his physical examination is unremarkable. His bilirubin is 15 mg/dl, Coombs test normal and peripheral blood smear unremarkable. The best medical management option is:

A. admit to hospital for double exchange transfusion
B. admit to hospital for observation
C. daily office visits checking bilirubin levels
D. office visit in 1 week and daily phone contact with family
E. home bilirubin phototherapy

35. Primitive or developmental reflexes include Moro, palmar (hand) grasp, rooting and asymmetric tonic neck. These reflexes should be extinct by:

A. 2 months of age
B. 4 months of age
C. 6 months of age
D. 9 months of age
E. 12 months of age

36–39. An 18-year-old woman comes in with polyuria, thirst, nausea and vomiting. On examination, she is clinically dehydrated, somnolent and tachypneic. Her urine is positive for glucose and ketones and her finger stix glucose is 250 mg/dl.

36. The most appropriate next step in her management is:

A. metformin
B. sulfonylurea
C. dietary advice
D. admission to hospital

37. The following are useful in the management of diabetic keto-acidosis (DKA) except:

A. intravenous fluid
B. insulin
C. potassium supplementation
D. oral hypoglycemic agents

38. All of the following can complicate the management of diabetes mellitus except:

A. prednisone
B. propranolol
C. bendrofluazide
D. non-steroidal anti-inflammatory drugs

39. The following are recognized complications of diabetes except:

A. retinopathy
B. nephropathy
C. osteoporosis
D. peripheral neuropathy
E. gastroparesis

40. The following are useful antianginal drugs except:

A. calcium channel blockers
B. nitrates
C. β-blockers
D. codeine and acetaminophen
E. aspirin

41. The following are useful in the management of asthma except:

A. β-blockers
B. steroids
C. β-receptor agonists
D. theophyllines

42. Which of the following is associated with dermatitis herpetiformis?

A. ulcerative colitis
B. celiac disease
C. diverticulosis
D. irritable bowel syndrome

43. Antimitochondrial antibodies are found in over 90% of which of the following conditions:

A. primary biliary cirrhosis
B. primary sclerosing cholangitis
C. lupus
D. pulmonary fibrosis

44. Which of the following is not associated with male infertility?

A. alcohol
B. sulfasalazine
C. XXY chromosomal pattern
D. sperm count of 50 million/ml

45–46. A 23-year-old white woman presents with three episodes of transient loss of vision in the right eye. All three episodes last for 2–3 days. In addition she also reports an episode 3 years ago when she developed weakness and numbness of her right arm which resolved after 1 week. On examination her visual acuity is 20/60 in her right eye and 20/20 in her left. The left optic disc is pale compared to the right. The only other significant finding was dysdiadachokinesia on the right side. You suspect that she has multiple sclerosis.

45. All the following are useful in establishing the diagnosis in MS except:

A. brain stem-evoked potentials
B. MRI
C. CSF oligoclonal bands
D. visual evoked responses
E. CT scan

46. The following have been shown to be efficacious treatments for MS except:

A. β-interferons
B. steroids copolymer 1
C. methotrexate
D. aspirin

47–48.   You see a 40-year-old businessman in your office who is complaining of intermittent dysphagia for solid foods that has been going on for years. He feels that sometimes the food 'gets stuck' and points to the region of the xyphoid. He denies having any problems with fluids and has no heartburn or regurgitation.

47.   The most likely diagnosis is:

A. achalasia
B. diffuse esophageal spasm
C. Schatzki's ring (lower esophageal rings)
D. esophageal carcinoma

48.   The test most likely to confirm the diagnosis is:

A. endoscopy with mucosal biopsy
B. esophageal manometry
C. barium swallow
D. 24-hour pH monitoring

49.   A 50-year-old woman is 5 weeks post-lumpectomy on her left breast for what proved to be a fibroadenoma. She returns to your office with complaints of burning pain and a mass on the lower outer quadrant of her left breast. The pain has been present for 1–2 days. On exam, you are able to able to palpate a cord-like mass approximately 2 cm long that is freely mobile in the subcutaneous tissue. There is some minimal skin dimpling around the mass. What is the most likely diagnosis?

A. recurrence of fibroadenoma
B. neoplasm
C. superficial thrombophlebitis
D. galactocele

50.   When measuring blood pressure the following can all cause erroneous elevated readings except:

A. narrow or too short cuff
B. loose cuff
C. if the brachial artery is at or above the heart during measurement
D. if the brachial artery is much below the heart during measurement

51.   Abrupt withdrawal of the following drugs can be hazardous except:

A. atenolol
B. warfarin
C. steroids
D. diazepam
E. anticonvulsants

Emergency room

52.   A 4-year-old is brought to the ER with a 6-hour history of high spiking fevers, and more recently drooling and difficulty swallowing. A cursory examination reveals a toxic and anxious-appearing child. The child is calm, sitting up with neck and chin extended. The only vocalization is an occasional muffled 'mommy'. The next step in diagnosis or management is:

A. remove child from the mother to auscultate lungs
B. examine the throat
C. obtain a chest radiograph
D. draw blood for culture and laboratory studies
E. remove child to operating room for anesthesia and intubation

53.   Paramedics bring a 4-year-old into the ER performing CPR. The child has a heart rate of 30 beats per minute, no pulses, is not spontaneously breathing, cool to the touch, and appears to be severely dehydrated. The child is receiving chest compressions, endotracheally intubated receiving bag ventilation with 100% oxygen, and receiving epinephrine and atropine via the endotracheal tube. A number of attempts at intravenous access have failed. The next step is to:

A. defibrillate at 2 J/kg
B. administer high-dose epinephrine via the endotracheal tube
C. obtain arterial blood gas
D. place a central venous cut-down for intravenous access
E. place an intraosseous needle

54.   Paramedics bring a 6-year-old to the ER. He smells strongly of smoke and his clothes are covered in soot. The paramedics state that he was in the house for quite a while before the firemen could remove him. He is currently receiving oxygen with a non-rebreather face mask. He is conscious, crying and asking for his mother. Physical examination reveals tachypnea, tachycardia and remarkably no burns and no soot in his upper airway. The initial combination of tests that should be obtained should include:

A. co-oximetry
B. carboxyhemoglobin, arterial blood gas and chest radiograph
C. arterial blood gas, carboxyhemoglobin, complete blood count, and chest radiograph
D. chest radiograph and arterial blood gas
E. no laboratory test required at this time, observe patient

55.   A 3-year-old has been visiting his grandparents for the past 6 hours. He has spent a lot of time playing in the basement in and around boxes of old clothes packed in mothballs.

He is brought to the emergency room because of a sudden onset of lethargy and irritability. On physical examination you have found pallor, jaundice, splenomegaly and noted that the urine in his diaper is red-tinged. You are concerned the child has a hemolytic anemia. The most likely diagnosis is:

A. autoimmune hemolytic anemia
B. hereditary spherocytosis
C. pyruvate kinase deficiency
D. glucose-6-phosphate dehydrogenase (G6PD) deficiency
E. paroxysmal nocturnal hemoglobinuria

56. An 18-year-old man was involved in a road traffic accident while cycling. On examination he is distressed and acutely dyspneic with a respiratory rate of 55 per minute and a pulse of 130. Breath sounds are diminished on the left side, and the chest is hyperresonant to percussion on that side. The most appropriate first step in his initial management is:

A. administer 100% oxygen
B. measure arterial blood gases before taking any further steps
C. order a chest X-ray
D. get an ECG
E. insert a wide bore needle in the second intercostal space in the mid-clavicular line on the left-hand side

57. You are asked to evaluate a patient involved in a brawl and found to have a possible blowout fracture of the right eye. All of the following are true regarding this condition except:

A. double vision
B. hypesthesia of the ipsilateral cheek and upper lip
C. restricted eye movement
D. crepitus (subcutaneous emphysema) on palpation of the eyelids
E. emergent orbital decompression to correct double vision

58–59. A 42-year-old woman attends the ER with a 2-day history of vomiting. She has had longstanding epigastric pain intermittently for the past 10 years. This pain was relieved by the frequent use of antacids. On examination there is marked tenderness and fullness in the epigastric area and visible peristalsis. Bowel sounds are normal; rectal examination is also normal.

58. The most likely diagnosis is:

A. colonic carcinoma
B. acute cholecystitis
C. gastric outlet obstruction
D. small bowel carcinoma
E. Crohn disease

59. The most likely metabolic imbalance expected in this patient is:

A. hypochloremic, hypokalemic metabolic alkalosis
B. hyperchloremic, hypokalemic metabolic alkalosis
C. hyperchloremic, hyperkalemic metabolic acidosis
D. hyperchloremic, hyperkalemic metabolic alkalosis

60. Oral rehydration therapy (ORT) is a mainstay for the treatment of dehydration in Third World countries. Families manage patients out of the hospital in a safe manner, with a success rate that matches that of parenteral rehydration in industrialized countries. The greatest obstacle to the acceptance of ORT in industrialized countries is:

A. health care providers
B. parents
C. patients
D. hospitals
E. insurance companies

61. An 18-month-old child is brought to the ER secondary to irritability, vomiting, colicky pain and bloody, mucous stools. Physical examination reveals a child that is pale and irritable, and on abdominal exam a sausage-shaped mass is palpable in the region of the ascending to transverse colon. The next management step is:

A. abdominal ultrasound
B. abdominal radiograph
C. barium enema
D. prompt pediatric surgical consultation
E. abdominal CT scan

62. The differential diagnosis of an adolescent female with right lower quadrant abdominal pain should include each of the following except:

A. ovarian torsion
B. appendicitis
C. ectopic tubal pregnancy
D. pelvic inflammatory disease
E. inflammatory bowel disease

63. For the pairs of drugs listed below, the former can be used to treat an overdose of the latter except:

A. acetylcysteine is used in the treatment of acetaminophen overdose
B. flumazenil is used in the treatment of barbiturate overdose
C. methylene blue is used in the treatment of methemoglobinemia caused by dapsone overdose
D. naloxone is used in the treatment of opioid overdose
E. ethanol can be used in treatment of methanol and ethylene glycol overdose

64–65.   A 19-year-old woman is referred for investigation of headaches. These had started 2 months previously and were worse in the mornings. She had previously been well, having visited her primary care physician previously only for treatment of severe acne. At that time the doctor had also given her contraceptive advice.

Examination showed her to be obese with an unsteady gait and some blurring of the optic disc margin. Visual acuity was 20/20. Her acne was very well controlled.

64.   The most appropriate initial investigation of this patient is:

A. CT and LP
B. MRI
C. visual field testing
D. toxicological screening

65.   Which one of the following does not precipitate pseudotumor cerebri?

A. retinoic acid
B. tetracycline
C. steroids
D. estrogens
E. acetazolamide

66.   An 18-year-old male with a history of supraventricular tachycardia is brought into the ER by the EMS. He is mumbling that his 'heart is racing'. He is disoriented and having difficulty breathing. Examination reveals a blood pressure of 64/30, a weak, rapid carotid pulse and pale, cool skin. The ECG shows a narrow-QRS tachycardia at 220 beats/min. The most appropriate initial management of this patient is:

A. intravenous administration of 2.5 mg of verapamil
B. administer sedation, then deliver synchronized countershock at 50 J
C. administer sedation, then deliver unsynchronized countershock at 100 J
D. reassess the patient's pulse, reconfirm the rhythm on the monitor and then proceed immediately with synchronized countershock at 200 J
E. intravenous adenosine at 6 mg

Hospital

67.   You are called to the ICU to certify brain death. Which of the following physical findings is inconsistent with brain stem death?

A. absent corneals
B. ankle jerks present
C. absent gag reflex
D. decerebrate posturing
E. absent pupillary reflexes

68.   You are called to see a patient who is complaining of shortness of breath. The nurse that is looking after the patient hands you the strip shown (Figure 6). The rhythm shown is:

A. atrial flutter with 2:1 block
B. first-degree heart block
C. atrial fibrillation
D. ventricular tachycardia
E. supraventricular tachycardia

69.   While being examined the patient starts to complain of shortness of breath, and feeling 'unwell'. His BP is 110/60. The following are all used in the management of atrial fibrillation except:

A. digoxin
B. heparin and warfarin
C. amiodarone
D. adenosine
E. procainamide

70.   A 55-year-old man is seen in the ER for chest pain. The rhythm strip is shown in Figure 7. What is the rhythm?

A. atrial fibrillation
B. atrial flutter
C. complete heart block
D. Mobitz 2:1 block

71.   Which of the following is NOT a formal indication for coronary artery bypass grafting (CABG)?

A. significant left main coronary artery disease
B. post-myocardial infarction angina
C. two-vessel disease involving proximal left anterior descending artery (LAD)
D. three-vessel disease involving proximal LAD
E. all of the above are indications

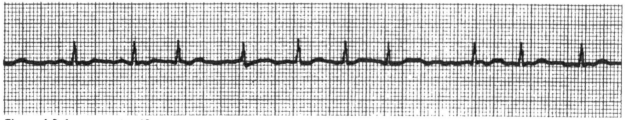

Figure 6 Refer to question 68

72. A 60-year-old widowed woman is admitted with thyrotoxicosis. On mental status examination she is disoriented to time and to place, is easily distracted and agitated, and has labile, tearful affect. Her recollection for three objects at 5 minutes is 0/3, and she cannot perform serial subtractions or reversed spelling. During the interview she talks to her husband (deceased) as if he were in the room, and some of her answers have bizarre content. Her relatives report that for several days before admission she has been very agitated and sleepless during the night. The most appropriate diagnosis is:

A. brief reactive psychosis
B. Alzheimer dementia
C. depression with psychotic features
D. delirium
E. Korsakoff dementia

73. A 35-year-old lawyer is referred to psychiatry before undergoing plastic surgery for his nose. He has a normally proportioned face, and his nose has no obvious abnormalities or deformities. He recognizes that most people see him as good-looking, but he complaints bitterly that the bridge of his nose is extremely large. He has recently quit going to court for his cases because he feels ridiculous and deformed, and reports spending a good deal of his time checking his nose in mirrors or store windows. He wears dark glasses at all times to hide his 'ugly' nose. The most likely diagnosis is:

A. factitious disorder
B. body dysmorphic disorder
C. simple phobia
D. conversion disorder
E. somatization disorder

74. You are called to the ER to see a 42-year-old, poorly controlled diabetic patient, complaining of double vision since waking up this morning. She was in her usual state of health until 2 days ago when she noted that she was having a low-grade fever, pain over her right cheek and nasal congestion accompanied by a thin bloody discharge, which she attributed to her old sinusitis. On physical examination, she has reduction of ocular motion, chemosis and proptosis of the right eye. The nasal turbinates look normal on the left and are dusky red on the right. The skin of her right cheek is

inflamed. A CT scan of her sinuses shows opacification of her right side. All of the following statements about this patient's management are true except:

A. she needs emergent referral for debridement of craniofacial lesions
B. amphotericin B needs to be started immediately
C. if she has an abnormal renal function ketoconazole is an acceptable alternative
D. isolation of the causative pathogen can be difficult

75. Which of the following statements about HIV-associated nephropathy (HIVAN) is true?

A. HIVAN is most common in white males
B. ultrasound examination reveals small kidneys
C. patients have high blood pressure that is difficult to control
D. there is rapid progression to ESRD without treatment
E. urinalysis shows minimal proteinuria

76. A 63-year-old male with hypertension and peripheral vasculopathy is post-operative day 10 after an abdominal aortic aneurysm (AAA) repair. Over the last 5 days he has had persistent fevers, spiking as high as 102.5°F this morning. He is noted on physical exam to have several small, scattered petechiae on his lower extremities bilaterally (right side greater than left). His blood pressure is 100/40, and his cardiac output is 8.2 l/min, with a cardiac index of 4.7. Blood cultures have grown 3/4 bottles of methicillin-resistant *Staphylococcus aureus* on two occasions in the last 4 days. Which of the following is the best method of management for this patient's condition?

A. excision and replacement of artificial graft with uninfected material
B. vancomycin and gentamicin for 30 days
C. excision of infected graft and axillobifemoral bypass
D. extra-anatomic aorto-aortic bypass

77. Your patient from the previous question recovers remarkably well thanks to your timely intervention. However, over the course of the next 2–3 days his urine output falls, and he is now in oliguric renal failure, making only

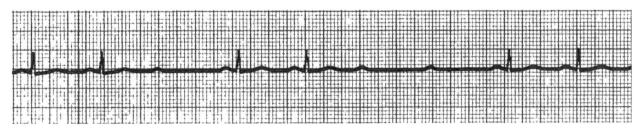

Figure 7 Refer to question 70

100 cc of urine in the last 24 hours, and only 20 in the last 8-hour shift. His BUN has risen from 17 mg/dl to 74 mg/dl, and what little urine he produces is darkly colored. Which of the following statements is FALSE about the pathophysiology of this patient's state?

A. back-leakage plays an important role
B. underperfusion of the kidneys was the most likely etiologic event
C. tubular obstruction and increased intratubular pressures play important roles
D. increased concentrations of urea in the blood is known to cause platelet dysfunction, encephalopathy, and immune system dysfunction

78. Your patient is a 47-year-old woman with stage IV breast CA, being treated with chemotherapy until 2 months ago. She is 5′7″ and over the last year her weight has dropped from 135 lb to 95 lb. Her chief presenting complaint is persistent nausea and vomiting, inability to tolerate any significant p.o. liquids or solids, and a sensation of distention. An obstruction series demonstrates no significant abnormalities, and a CT scan shows dilated first, second and proximal third segments of the duodenum. What is the most appropriate test to confirm her diagnosis?

A. ERCP
B. EGD
C. barium swallow
D. angiography

79. Your patient is a male neonate who presented shortly after birth with coughing, respiratory distress and excessive drooling. He is afebrile with an HR of 220, RR of 34 and blood pressure of 82/44. An attempt to pass a nasogastric tube meets resistance and no return of gastric fluid. Posterior–anterior and lateral X-rays confirm the diagnosis showing a blind proximal pouch. Which of the following statements is FALSE regarding tracheo-esophageal fistulas (TEFs)?

A. the most common type is a blind-ending proximal esophagus with a distal TEF
B. there is an association between TEFs and trisomy 21 (Down syndrome)
C. there is a significant male preponderance
D. gastroesophageal reflux is a common complication

80–81. You are asked to see a patient in the ICU with low blood pressure despite being on dopamine. You consider dobutamine.

80. Which one of the following statements about dobutamine is incorrect?

A. it stimulates dopaminergic receptors
B. it decreases peripheral vascular resistance
C. it is a synthetic sympathomimetic amine and is useful in the treatment of heart failure
D. it has both β-1 and α-adrenergic receptor stimulating effects
E. it increases renal perfusion by increasing cardiac output

81. There is minimal improvement in the BP with dobutamine. You are now considering norepinephrine infusion. Which of the following statements regarding norepinephrine is incorrect?

A. norepinephrine induces renal and mesenteric vasoconstriction
B. norepinephrine has both β-1 and α-adrenergic effects
C. norepinephrine decreases myocardial oxygen demand and should be considered early in the management of patients with ischemic heart disease
D. ischemic necrosis and sloughing of superficial tissues may result from extravasation of norepinephrine
E. norepinephrine has minimal β-2 effect

82–83. Two months prior to an admission, a 66-year-old woman presented to her primary care physician with a 1-month history of malaise. In the preceding week she had experienced ache in her nose and under the right eye. A clinical diagnosis of sinusitis was made and she was given a course of amoxicillin. This brought no significant relief. In the 10 days before admission she had become increasingly tired and nauseated. On the day before admission she had become breathless and coughed up a small amount of blood. She had not smoked for 20 years and drank no alcohol. She took no regular medication. She had two daughters, one of whom suffered from rheumatoid arthritis. On examination, she was afebrile, her pulse was 100/min and regular, and her blood pressure was 145/90 mmHg. Her jugular venous pressure was not raised and she had no dependent edema. Heart sounds were normal with no added sounds or murmurs. There were bilateral coarse crackles in both lungs. She had left foot drop and right wrist drop. The urine contained blood (+++) on urinalysis. CT of the head showed marked thickening of the sinus membranes with air-fluid levels. Chest X-ray showed bilateral diffuse alveolar shadowing; and normal heart size.

Initial investigations:

Plasma Na⁺	140 mmol/l
Plasma K⁺	6.6 mmol/l
Plasma urea	45 mmol/l
Plasma creatinine	3.4 mg/dl

82. The likely diagnosis is:

A. rheumatoid arthritis
B. sarcoidosis
C. Wegener granulomatosis
D. diabetes mellitus
E. Goodpasture syndrome

83. Which antibody will be the most helpful in the diagnosis?

A. pANCA
B. cANCA
C. anti-GBM antibodies
D. antimitochondrial antibodies

84. You are unable to obtain intravenous access in a patient with pulseless electrical activity. Advanced cardiac life support medications that may be administered via the endotracheal tube include:

A. lidocaine, epinephrine, atropine
B. lidocaine, furosemide, amiodarone
C. lidocaine, atropine, sodium bicarbonate, bretylium
D. epinephrine, sodium bicarbonate, calcium chloride, magnesium

85–87. A 15-year-old Indian girl presents with increasing malaise and vomiting. She is a recent immigrant to the USA. Her past medical history is remarkable only for TB as a child. On examination, her blood pressure was 82/55, and her heart rate was 80. The rest of the examination was unremarkable except for dark mucous membranes and dark palmar creases.

Investigations show:

Plasma Na$^+$	127 mmol/l
Plasma K$^+$	5.7 mmol/l
Plasma urea	14 mg/l
Plasma creatinine	1.2 mg/dl
Plasma bicarbonate	13 mmol/l
Plasma glucose	50 mg/dl

She was given medication to help with the nausea and vomiting. A few minutes afterwards she was unable to speak, her eyes deviated upwards and her neck extended and became rigid.

85. The most appropriate immediate management of this patient is:

A. intramuscular haloperidol
B. intravenous diazepam
C. intramuscular benztropine
D. intravenous calcium chloride
E. intravenous 50% dextrose

86. What is the most likely cause of the initial presentation?

A. adrenocortical deficiency
B. diabetic keto-acidosis
C. hypothyroidism
D. hyperthyroidism

87. The most appropriate initial treatment for this patient is:

A. intravenous thyroxine
B. intravenous fluids and cortisol
C. carbimazole
D. intravenous glucose

88–89. A 29-year-old black female complains of a painful red eye which came on overnight. She also gives a history of shortness of breath which she attributed to her asthma. On examination, she has anterior uveitis and painful red circumscribed lesions on her shins. You suspect sarcoidosis.

88. Appropriate initial tests in the evaluation of this woman include all of the following except:

A. chest X-ray
B. serum angiotensin-converting enzyme levels
C. Kveim test
D. biopsy of the skin lesion

89. All of the following are recognized complications of sarcoid except:

A. hypopituitarism
B. seizures
C. dyspnea
D. peripheral neuropathy
E. inflammatory bowel disease

90. A 35-year-old female employee of the local power company arrives in the trauma bay after sustaining a high-voltage burn to her right arm and leg. Her immediate recovery is uncomplicated, and she is able to leave the hospital on post-admission day 4. Which of the following is NOT a characteristic long-term complication of her electrocution injury?

A. cholelithiasis
B. cataract formation
C. delayed hemorrhage
D. pituitary dysfunction

91–92. A 54-year-old woman was admitted with a sudden onset of pain in the right iliac fossa radiating to her right thigh which was worse on movement. The pain continued and she had difficulty in walking. She had had rheumatic fever as a child and was later diagnosed as having mitral stenosis. She had a mitral valve replacement 4 years previously and was on warfarin and digoxin. On examination she had a temperature of 99.6°F, a pulse of 80/min, irregularly irregular, and a blood pressure of 125/96 in both arms. The apex was slightly to the left of the midclavicular line. A mid-diastolic murmur was heard at that apex and a systolic murmur with valve clicking was heard over the precordium. Lungs were clear. Initially there were no focal abnormal neurologic signs but over a period of 2 days her right knee reflex was found to be absent and she developed an area of anesthesia over the anterior right thigh and medial aspect of her right leg. Peripheral pulses were intact. An abdominal X-ray was normal apart from a calcified mass to the right of the midline thought to be a lymph node. A lumbar spine X-ray was normal.

Investigations:
Hb	9.1 g/dl
WBC	9×10^9/l
Erythrocyte sedimentation rate	1 mm/h

91. The likely cause of her symptoms is:

A. ruptured aortic aneurysm
B. retroperitoneal hemorrhage
C. pelvic tumor
D. Guillain–Barré syndrome (GBS)

92. While in hospital, warfarin was initially discontinued. However, prior to discharge the decision was made to restart her anticoagulation. She was started on heparin but unfortunately developed severe rectal bleeding 2 hours after starting. Which of the following agents will reverse the anticoagulant effect of heparin?

A. vitamin K
B. desferrioxamine
C. factor VIII
D. protamine sulfate

Other encounters

93. Increased urinary pH favors the formation of which of the following stones:

A. calcium oxalate stones
B. cysteine stones
C. struvite stones
D. uric acid stones

94. All of the following are contraindications for administration of thrombolytic therapy except:

A. age over 80
B. active bleeding
C. history of cerebral aneurysm
D. surgery 7 days prior to infarction
E. active inflammatory bowel disease

95. Malignant (invasive) otitis externa is usually caused by:

A. *Haemophilus influenzae*
B. *Moraxella catarrhalis*
C. *Streptococcus pneumoniae*
D. *Staphylococcus aureus*
E. *Pseudomonas aeruginosa*

96. You are interested in studying the effect of smoking tobacco on psoriasis. In the course of designing a study, you notice that many of the patients who smoke also use alcohol, which has already been shown to have an effect on this disease. This problem is known as:

A. interference
B. recall bias
C. confounding
D. misclassification
E. none of the above

97. You are interested in studying the association between computer terminal use and birth defects. You design a study in which you question 100 patients with children who had some type of birth defect and 100 controls with normal children. A major concern in designing this study is:

A. selection bias
B. recall bias
C. confounding
D. misclassification
E. none of the above

98. A 43-year-old woman presents to your office complaining of vaginal spotting. The patient is concerned that she may have uterine cancer and asks you how common this type of cancer is in women her age. You refer to a reference text which includes data on both the incidence and prevalence of endometrial cancer in women aged 40–45. The problem with providing the patient with the prevalence data from this text is that:

A. the group of patients in your text may not reflect the population from which your patient is derived
B. these data would include women who acquired endometrial cancer prior to age 40
C. these data may not include data on women who acquired endometrial cancer after age 40 but died prior to the time that this study was conducted
D. A and B
E. all of the above

99. You are interested in studying patient survival after treatment for laryngeal carcinoma. Utilizing a large extant database, you find that the probability of survival after 1 year of disease is *x* and that the probability of survival after

2 years of disease, given that the patient already survived to 1 year, is y. In order to estimate the overall survival after 2 years, you consult with a statistician who advises you that the survival after 2 years $= xy$. The statistician most probably computed this number utilizing:

A. Wilcoxon rank–sum coefficient
B. Kaplan–Meier estimator of survival
C. two-way analysis of variance
D. logistic regression
E. none of the above

TEST THREE: ANSWERS

1. **Answer: A**

The key features of fetal alcohol syndrome are microcephaly, short palpebral fissures, smooth philtrum, and a thin, smooth upper lip. There are often maxillary hypoplasia, prominent ears and microphthalmia. The features do vary, related to the amount of alcohol consumed during the pregnancy. There is often borderline to moderate mental retardation and hyperactivity present.

Reference: Zitelli and Davis, p. 24; Oski *et al.*, p. 2185

2. **Answer: C**

Developmental assessment is an important part of any physical examination in a child. A child typically pulls to a stand between 6 and 12 months, stands alone at 9–16 months, and walks three steps alone at 9–17 months. A 15-month-old can grasp a writing implement and scribble, and will imitate vertical or circular strokes at 24 months. An 18-month-old can stack two blocks, while a 24-month-old can stack six blocks. In speech development a 9–12 month old will use a few words, but mostly gestures, a 12–18-month-old uses 20–50 words, and an 18–24-month-old uses two-word sentences. That places the best estimate of this child's appropriate age at 18 months.

Reference: Zitelli and Davis, pp. 47–60

3. **Answer: E**

The most important risk factor is a positive family history. Incidence of breast cancer increases with age. Early menarche, late menopause and nulliparity increase the risk of breast cancer. Atypical lobular or ductal hyperplasia also increases the risk. Exposure to ionizing radiation, long-term postmenopausal hormone replacement therapy and alcohol consumption increase the risk.

Reference: Hortobagyi

4. **Answer: B**

Thyroid nodularity is very uncommon in this age range, and its presence in very young or very old patients increases the likelihood of malignancy. While nodules occur more frequently in females, the proportion of malignant to benign nodules is higher in males. The presence of a single nodule (4.7%) or a single nodule in a background of multinodularity

(4.1%) has a greater risk of malignancy than simple multinodularity with no dominant nodule. Note that the background nodularity does NOT increase the risk of malignancy. Family history of either papillary or medullary thyroid CA is a significant risk factor.

Reference: Sabiston, p. 1237

5. **Answer: B**

Regardless of the clinical presentation, a fine needle aspiration is the most appropriate method for distinguishing between a benign and a malignant histology. The FNA is not always definitive, but it can make a conclusive diagnosis in the most common class of thyroid cancer; papillary carcinomas have characteristic cleft nuclei on histologic exam. It is impossible, however, to determine adenomatous vs. carcinomatous histology of follicular cell tumors without a tissue sample (invasion beyond capsule is the hallmark). Anaplastic and medullary carcinomas are much less common – 4% and 1% respectively. Most patients with thyroid carcinoma have normal levels of thyroid hormone, and TSH level is therefore not helpful. A radioactive thyroid scan demonstrating a cold nodule would not be likely to alter your course of action.

Reference: Schlumberger

6. **Answer: E**

Nasal polyps are felt to be a result of recurrent infection or chronic inflammatory processes. They are unusual in children under 10 years of age, except in those with cystic fibrosis. Between 6 and 24% of patients with cystic fibrosis develop nasal polyps. Patients with atopy generally develop them at a later age. Any pediatric patient with nasal polyps should undergo a sweat chloride test; this is regardless of whether the patient has any respiratory or gastrointestinal symptoms. A chest radiograph and sputum culture may be useful if the patient is ultimately diagnosed with cystic fibrosis. Nasal cultures are generally not useful in treating sinusitis as many of the infections are mixed flora. Radiographs of the sinuses are not necessary if a CT scan of the sinuses is obtained.

Reference: Zitelli and Davis, pp. 701–2; Oski *et al.*, p. 1493

7. **Answer: B**

Encopresis or functional constipation is a diagnosis that may be made in older children, previously toilet trained, and without organic pathology. Psychologic symptoms are often present, or a previous history of an anal fissure that had caused pain on defecation. Most commonly there is associated recurrent abdominal pain often localized to the periumbilical region. The stools are often very large in caliber, and the incontinence is usually late in the afternoon to early evening. Occasionally, poor growth and decreased appetite are associated. Anterior displacement of the anus usually presents at an earlier age; when present, there is not a functional anal sphincter, resulting in incontinence. The barium enema rules out Hirschsprung disease, as the anal verge is not dilated in Hirschsprung's since its innervation is from a different source. Inflammatory bowel disease in the face of a normal white blood cell count and normal erythrocyte sedimentation rate is highly unlikely. A normal neurologic examination makes spina bifida occulta or tethered cord syndromes very unlikely.

Reference: Oski *et al.*, pp. 1843–5

8.   Answer: C

In HIV the only live vaccine that is contraindicated at this time is the oral polio vaccine (OPV), with the inactivated polio virus (IPV) being recommended. This recommendation may change as more data are collected. In all other forms of congenitally inherited forms of immunodeficiency or that related to malignancy and chemotherapy, live viral vaccinations are not recommended.

Reference: Oski *et al.*, pp. 612–33

9.   Answer: D

Gum hyperplasia is a side-effect of phenytoin. Rash, neutropenia, diplopia and ataxia are all recognized side-effects of carbamazepine.

Reference: Leppik, p. 125

10.   Answer: B

Coarctation of the aorta often presents as an incidental finding on a complete physical examination. The children are usually asymptomatic and without complaints. Often there is a systolic murmur on cardiac examination. Once the diagnosis is entertained referral to a pediatric cardiologist is immediately appropriate. Once the diagnosis is confirmed, surgical correction should ensue as appropriate. A coarctation that causes a palpable difference in blood pressure may result in left ventricular hypertrophy, which may be problematic if the coarctation is not corrected.

Reference: Oski *et al.*, pp. 1575–8

11.   Answer: E

The combination treatment of amoxicillin and clavulanic acid is useful clinically. The β–lactam inhibitors such as clavulanic acid, tazobactum and sulbactam have weak antibacterial activity but in combination therapy, and have been particularly useful against staphylococcal, streptococcal and

Haemophilus influenzae. Both metronidazole and nitrofurantoin cause peripheral neuropathy. Tetracycline should be avoided in pregnant women and children owing to the possibility of its causing discoloration of teeth and being deposited in bone. The aminoglycosides, such as gentamicin, cause ototoxicity and nephropathy.

Reference: Kelley, pp. 1843–54

12.   Answer: E

This young patient presents with a history typical of mild uveitis (inflammation of the anterior uveal tissue including the iris and ciliary body). The absence of a recent upper respiratory infection and epiphora with unilateral involvement over 2 weeks' duration makes viral conjunctivitis unlikely. Absence of itching of both eyes also places allergic conjunctivitis low on the list. Though bacterial conjunctivitis involves one eye, the absence of a mucopurulent discharge makes this diagnosis unlikely. Acute glaucoma usually presents unilaterally with a mid-dilated pupil, corneal edema, pain and moderate photophobia. The presence of a meiotic (small) pupil with a history of arthritis is consistent with uveitis. The inflammation results from a breakdown of the blood aqueous barrier with resultant increase in vascular permeability and exudation of both protein and white blood cells. Chronic low-grade inflammation can result in adhesions between the pupil and the lens posterior to it resulting in a fixed constricted pupil. Although a majority of cases of anterior uveitis are idiopathic, a number of etiologies can give rise to this presentation including ankylosing spondylitis, inflammatory bowel disease, Lyme disease, Reiter syndrome, collagen vascular diseases (e.g. systemic lupus) and Behçet disease. Juvenile rheumatoid arthritis is a leading etiology of uveitis in childhood.

Reference: Friedman *et al.*, pp. 181–3

13.   Answer: E

Chronic administration of steroids can, in addition to slow wound healing, result in all of the choices listed except optic neuritis. An increase in intraocular pressure has been reported in up to 30% of the general population using topical steroids for 4–6 weeks. Steroids can exacerbate a herpetic infection if viral shedding occurs at the time of use. They are useful in treating patients with giant cell arteritis and optic neuritis.

Reference: Wilson, pp. 381–2

14.   Answer: E

Episodes of transient visual loss (amaurosis fugax) in an elderly patient require an embolic workup including a complete cardiovascular evaluation to evaluate for arrhythmias, valvular and carotid-occlusive disease, assessment of retinal emboli on fundus exam and assessment for vertebrobasilar insufficiency. A 2% 1-year risk of cerebrovascular accident has been noted.

Reference: Friedman *et al.*, pp. 383–4

15. Answer: C

In the visual pathway, the optic chiasm is the site where nasal fibers (subserving the temporal visual field) cross the midline to join the temporal fibers (subserving the nasal visual field) from the opposite eye to form the contralateral optic tract. The chiasm lies in close proximity to the pituitary lobe located superiorly. Any expanding lesions such as non-secreting pituitary adenomas can compress each of the nasal fibers, resulting in the respective temporal visual fields being compromised. Patients will express this condition by noting loss of visual field to the sides. This type of visual field loss arises from the unique anatomy of the optic chiasm, and occurs nowhere else in the visual pathway. Although craniopharyngiomas can also present similarly, they usually occur in children. All lesions posterior to the optic chiasm will result in homonymous hemianopias (loss of visual field in both eyes involving either the right or left half).

Reference: Vander and Gault, p. 221

16. Answer: D

Homonymous hemianopic visual field defects occur posterior to the chiasm. Inferior fibers (that subserve the superior visual field) in the visual pathway anatomically loop around the temporal lobe. Lesions in this area give rise to a characteristic 'pie in the sky' homonymous visual field defect. Associated symptoms of such patients include formed hallucinations and *déjà vu* experiences. A 'pie on the floor' defect is associated with parietal lesions. Unformed hallucinations are associated with occipital lobe lesions.

Reference: Berson, pp. 114–17; Vander and Gault, pp. 24–5

17. Answer: E

Although the patient is instilling a β-blocker topically, systemic side-effects can occur. Drainage of tears and topical medical drops through the nasolacrimal duct system can result in systemic absorption by the nasal mucosa, a highly vascularized area. This route bypasses the hepatic circulation and is akin to intravenous administration. Beta-blockers are known to exacerbate asthma and depression, decrease heart rate, decrease libido and cause syncope. Deaths from topical β-blockers have been reported due to pulmonary complications. The most appropriate step would be to discontinue the drops and reassess the patient a few weeks later when the medication is completely washed out of the body.

Reference: Berson, pp. 137–8; Wilson, pp. 383–4

18. Answer: D

A subconjunctival hemorrhage presents typically with sudden onset and no other associated symptoms such as decreased vision, eye pain or discharge. It can be associated with a Valsalva maneuver such as sneezing, vomiting, coughing or straining. Inquiry should be made if the patient is using anticoagulants such as aspirin or warfarin and the blood pressure should be checked for evidence of hypertension. In the absence of trauma, reassurance and placebo therapy with artificial tears is all that is necessary. Spontaneous clearing occurs usually in 1–2 weeks. Kaposi sarcoma can mimic a subconjunctival hemorrhage, but the characteristic presentation noted above enables one to differentiate from this entity.

Reference: Cullom and Chang, pp. 119–20

19. Answer: B

Endotracheal intubation provides many advantages. These include the reduction of aspiration risk, permits suctioning of the trachea, ensures delivery of high concentration of oxygen, allows route of administration of some drugs and ensures delivery of adequate lung ventilation. It should only be attempted by trained individuals.

Reference: Cummins, p. 2.3

20. Answer: C

CAIs account for a number of side-effects including kidney stones, paresthesias, depression, anorexia, decreased libido, altered taste of carbonated soft drinks and hypokalemia. Patients known to have sulfonamide allergies should avoid them. A rare side-effect, aplastic anemia, has been reported with CAIs.

Reference: Wilson, p. 384

21. Answer: E

All the answers present with anisocoria (unevenly-sized pupils) with the exception of RAPD. Unilateral use of either a dilating drop (e.g. atropine) or a miotic (e.g. pilocarpine) can result in pharmacologic alteration of the pupil. Trauma involving the iris sphincter muscle can affect the muscle tone with pupillary dilation. In working up patients with uneven pupils, the size should be noted both in lit and dim settings. Physiologic anisocoria results in a pupillary size difference that does not change with light settings. In Horner syndrome the size difference is greater in dim light, pointing to a defect in the sympathetic innervation of the pupil. In Adie's pupil the opposite is the case, with a large discrepancy in bright light indicative of a defect in the parasympathetic innervation of the pupil. Damage to the efferent system results in anisocoria. In RAPD, the afferent system is involved. The swinging flashlight test enables one to test the pupillary response to direct light stimulus. Though one pupil constricts less compared to the other, both pupils are of the same size when the affected eye is directly stimulated since it perceives a dimmer light than the normal. What accounts for equal size of the pupils is the equal projection of ipsilateral pupillomotor fibers to both nuclei that control pupillary constriction. Direct stimulation of the unaffected eye results in greater pupillary constriction in both eyes. The relative size of the pupils indicates a difference in the response of the pupils to light stimulation.

Reference: Samuels and Feske, pp. 63–8

22. Answer: B

Parents are commonly concerned with repeated emesis with feeding. When the child's growth parameters are appropriate for age and the child's physical examination is normal the most important recommendation a pediatrician can offer is ongoing support and reassurance that this is normal. In such cases it is often helpful to observe the mother feeding the infant during the office visit. Although parents will often change formulas on their own, this is rarely the cause of spitting up.

Reference: Oski *et al.*, pp. 601–6

23. Answer: D

Nodulocystic lesions are the most severe in acne and are potentially scarring. Acne that is progressive, scarring or cystic should be referred to a dermatologist for a more aggressive therapeutic approach. Most acne can be successfully treated with topical medications. Topical therapy in conjunction with systemic antibiotics may be necessary in patients with a large inflammatory component.

Reference: Zitelli and Davis, pp. 241–2; Oski *et al.*, pp. 795–7

24. Answer: B

High sodium and high chloride are the classic findings on sweat testing. The levels of sodium and chloride are greater than 60 mmol. Seventy per cent of European patients have a mutation of the *DF508* gene which encodes a protein that sits on top of epithelial cells and controls transport of sodium, chloride and hence water across the cell. Other organs also produce thick secretions.

Reference: Kelley, pp. 2003–7

25. Answer: E

About 20% present with meconium ileus, a form of bowel obstruction. Malabsorption and diabetes are a result of pancreatic failure and bronchiectasis results from prolonged, recurrent chest infections. Hypothyroidism is not associated with cystic fibrosis.

Reference: Kelley, pp. 2003–7

26. Answer: C

Cystic fibrosis exhibits autosomal recessive inheritance and so statistically one in four offspring will be affected. There is variable penetrance and some are only mildly affected. Males and females are equally affected.

Reference: Kelley, pp. 2003–7

27. Answer: E

A manic episode is a distinct period during which there is an abnormally and persistently elevated, expansive or irritable mood, lasting at least one week. This change in mood is associated with inflated self-esteem or grandiosity, decreased need for sleep, pressured speech, flight of ideas, distractibility, increased involvement in goal-directed activities or psychomotor agitation, and/or increased involvement in pleasurable activities with a high potential for painful consequences. Delusions, hallucinations, lability of mood and violent behavior are common. Symptoms like those seen in a manic episode can be due to the direct effects of antidepressant medication, electroconvulsive therapy, light therapy, or medications prescribed for other medical conditions, in particular corticosteroids. Such presentations are not considered manic episodes and do not count towards the diagnosis of bipolar disorder, in spite of the fact that some evidence suggests that these patients are more likely to develop true manic episodes in the future.

Reference: DSM–IV, pp. 328–9

28. Answer: D

The essential characteristic of melancholia is pervasive anhedonia (i.e. loss of pleasure in all, or almost all, activities), or a lack of reactivity (or even a transient mood improvement) to usually pleasurable stimuli. In addition, a distinct quality of the depressed mood, circadian rhythm such that symptoms are usually worse in the morning, early morning awakening, prominent psychomotor changes (either agitation or retardation), significant anorexia or weight loss, and inappropriate guilt are commonly present. Leaden paralysis is not a feature of melancholia, but of atypical depression.

Reference: DSM–IV, pp. 383–4

29. Answer: E

Atypical features of major depression are defined by the presence of mood reactivity (i.e. the patient's mood brightens in response to positive events), associated with significant weight gain or increase in appetite, hypersomnia, leaden paralysis, or a longstanding pattern of interpersonal rejection sensitivity (which has resulted in significant social or occupational impairment at times when the patient is not depressed). These features are 2–3 times more common in women, and tend to occur in younger patients who have a more chronic course. These patients also commonly have marked somatic anxiety symptoms, and are usually seen first by a cardiologist. Patients with atypical depression are more likely to respond to MAOIs, in particular if they have a history of panic attacks.

Reference: DSM–IV, pp. 384–5; Winokur and Clayton, p. 372

30. Answer: E

Binge eating is a prominent feature of both anorexia and bulimia nervosa. Kleine–Levin syndrome, or periodic somnolence and bulimia, is an episodic disorder characterized by periods of days or weeks during which the patients, mostly adolescent boys, sleep 8 or more hours a day, awakening just long enough to eat and attend to toilet activities. During the episodes the patients appear dull, confused, restless and troubled by hallucinations. The cause is unknown, and the disorder tends to disappear in adult life. Bilateral mesial temporal lobe lesions can cause a human analog of Klüver–Bucy syndrome, with placidity (i.e. lack of response to stimuli), bulimia, amnesia, aphasia or dementia.

Reference: DSM–IV, pp. 539–40, 546–8; Adams *et al.*, pp. 362, 453; Hales and Yudofsky, pp. 781–2

31. Answer: B

Fat necrosis is usually found over a bony prominence and may be secondary to pressure or trauma during delivery. Most lesions resolve spontaneously, and require no intervention. Occasionally, a lesion may develop a calcification and require surgery.

Reference: Zitelli and Davis, p. 37

32. Answer: D

The perianal tape test is the preferred method of diagnosing pinworms, *Enterobius vermicularis*. This is a common helminthic parasite of humans and is distributed worldwide, affecting all socioeconomic groups. Typically children become infected with it after ingesting eggs deposited on perianal skin. During the life cycle the mature pregnant females migrate to the perianal skin and deposit their eggs. This is a very infectious agent and once diagnosed all members of a household should be treated. The gastric string test is utilized in diagnosing *Giardia lamblia*. Stool for leukocyte and culture is useful in diagnosing bacterial etiologies of gastroenteritis. Stool for ova and parasite can be used to make this diagnosis but is time-consuming and expensive. The perianal tape test can be performed in any office with a low-powered microscope.

Reference: Zitelli and Davis, pp. 547–8; Oski *et al.*, pp. 1408–9

33. Answer: A

Children 3 years old and younger are at a higher risk for child abuse. Other known factors include parental alcoholism, addiction or psychosis, foster children and adopted children, infants born with congenital anomalies and children with chronic illness.

Reference: Zitelli and Davis, pp. 133–4; Oski *et al.*, pp. 650–4

34. Answer: C

Management of breast milk jaundice tends to be conservative, especially if the neonate has no known risk factors. This child falls into this category with no evidence of hemolysis on peripheral blood smear and a normal Coombs test. A level of 15 mg/dl warrants close monitoring but no active intervention at this time. Given the child's age it should decline on its own in the next day or two. If it were to increase over 20 mg/dl most pediatricians would initiate phototherapy.

Even levels as high as 30 mg/dl are starting to be tolerated (in hospital) without exchange transfusion unless the child has symptoms or has risk factors.

Reference: Oski *et al.*, pp. 446–54

35. Answer: C

The primitive or developmental reflexes are involuntary reflexes that indicate the integrated activity of multiple muscle groups. As the child gets older and higher cortical function develops there is more voluntary control and muscular flexion and extension become balanced.

Reference: Zitelli and Davis, pp. 47–9; Oski *et al.*, pp. 305–6

36. Answer: D

This woman has diabetic keto-acidosis and needs to be admitted to hospital. She is volume depleted, ketonemic and hyperglycemic. She is also probably acidotic as evidenced by the tachypnea.

Reference: Kelley, pp. 2164–5

37. Answer: D

The basis of management of DKA is aggressive fluid replacement, insulin to treat the hyperglycemia and potassium supplementation to avoid hypokalemia. There is no place for oral hypoglycemic agents.

Reference: Kelley, pp. 2164–5

38. Answer: D

Prednisone and bendrofluazide increase blood glucose levels and can complicate mangement of diabetes. Beta-blockers, especially if non-selective, can mask the patient's awareness of hypoglycemia and should be avoided if possible. NSAIDs have no effect on glycemic control.

Reference: Rudy and Kurowski, pp. 513–41

39. Answer: C

Retinopathy, nephropathy, gastroparesis and peripheral neuropathy are all complications of diabetes and progression is related to control. There is no link between osteoporosis and diabetes.

Reference: Rudy and Kurowski, pp. 333, 513–41

40. Answer: D

Nitrates, β-blockers and calcium channel blockers are all frontline medications in the treatment of angina. Codeine and acetaminophen have no place in the management of angina. Aspirin, although not strictly an antianginal, is efficacious in primary and secondary prevention of MI.

Reference: Kelley, p. 321

41. Answer: A

Beta-blockers will exacerbate asthma by causing bronchoconstriction and are contraindicated. Short and long-acting β-adrenergic receptor agonists alone or in combination with anticholinergic agents such as ipratropium are effective bronchodilators. The methylxanthines such as theophylline are also useful agents but the narrow therapeutic index has limited their use. Inhaled and systemic steroids are the most effective agents in controlling asthma.

Reference: Kelley, pp. 1978–9

42. Answer: B

Dermatitis herpetiformis, a pruritic papulovesicular rash, typically occurs over the elbows, buttocks, shoulders and knees, is highly specific and is found in patients with celiac disease. Diverticulosis and irritable bowel syndrome are not associated with skin lesions. Ulcerative colitis does not cause dermatitis herpetiformis but is associated with pyoderma gangrenosum.

Reference: Kelley, pp. 723–4

43. Answer: A

Antimitochondrial antibodies are found in over 90% of patients with primary biliary cirrhosis. Lupus, pulmonary fibrosis and primary sclerosing cholangitis are not associated with antimitochondrial antibodies.

Reference: Kelley, p. 660

44. Answer: D

About 15% of couples in the US are infertile and in 30% of these, the male has the primary abnormality contributing to the infertility. Sperm counts of 50 million/ml or higher are considered normal. Alcohol and sulfasalazine are associated with hypofertility. XXY individuals are infertile.

Reference: Kelley, pp. 2151–3, 2235

45. Answer: E

CT is the least useful test for diagnosing MS. Characteristic findings on MRI showing demyelination, together with visual evoked responses and oligoclonal bands are the most widely used tests. However, the history and physical examination together with characteristic MRI findings may be all that is needed in the hands of an experienced neurologist. Brain stem-evoked potentials may also be useful in some cases. Double contrast CT may be useful for patients who cannot have MRI.

Reference: Samuels and Feske, p. 351

46. Answer: D

Beta-interferons have received much attention and have been shown to decrease the frequency and severity of relapses. Steroids can reduce the severity of the attack but do not appear to have an effect on disability. Small trials with copolymer 1 and methotrexate have also been shown to reduce the severity of attacks. Aspirin does not appear to have an effect on the progression of MS.

Reference: Samuels and Feske, p. 351

47–48. Answers: D (47), C (48)

Lower esophageal rings at the squamocolumnar junction can cause intermittent dysphagia when the diameter of the ring is less than 12 mm. They can give rise to intermittent bolus impaction. These patients have long symptom-free intervals, which with time become shortened, until eventually symptoms are continuous. The diagnosis is made on barium swallow. Dilatation with bougies is curative. Esophageal spasm is characterized by dysphagia for solids as well as liquids, and can be exacerbated by cold liquids. Achalasia causes a motor-type dysphagia, associated with regurgitation, occasional chest pain and weight loss. Esophageal cancer is characterized by a mechanical–progressive dysphagia.

Reference: Dornbrand et al., pp. 196–200

49. Answer: C

Mondor disease is a relatively rare condition consisting of thrombophlebitis of a superficial vein leading away from the surface of the breast. This condition may develop 4–6 weeks after any type of breast surgery, or after strenuous exercise, although many cases have no known etiology. Patients often notice the phlebitis when moving or stretching the overlying skin. The problem is generally self-limited, and will usually disappear on its own. In this case, given the benign histology, the index of suspicion for carcinoma is low, but in cases where the level of suspicion is higher, mammography may be indicated. The only necessary treatment is careful warmth, although some physicians will prescribe NSAIDs. Fibroadenoma recurrence is unlikely in this time span, as is the development of a new neoplasm. A galactocele is highly unlikely in a woman who is not postpartum.

Reference: Greenfield, pp. 1377–8

50. Answer: C

It is important that a correctly fitting cuff is used when taking BP measurements. In addition, the brachial artery should be at the level of the heart during measurements. A loose or narrow cuff or if the brachial artery is too much below the heart will give falsely high readings.

Reference: Bates, p. 272

51. Answer: B

Abrupt withdrawal of β-blockers can cause tachycardia hypertension and can exacerbate myocardial ischemia. Sudden withdrawal of steroids can cause adrenocortical crisis. Seizures can be precipitated by sudden withdrawal of anticonvulsants. Sudden withdrawal of benzodiazepines can cause agitation, anxiety and seizures. Warfarin can be stopped abruptly.

Reference: Cummins, pp. 8.11–8.12; Sprigings et al., p. 272; Leppik, pp. 166–7

52. Answer: E

Epiglottitis is an emergent form of upper airway obstruction. This is a potentially life-threatening bacterial infection. The glottic opening is acutely narrowed by cellulitis and edema of the epiglottis, aryepiglottic folds, and hypopharynx. Management of the airway is the initial consideration, prior to obtaining laboratory studies or initiating antibiotics. Owing to the risk of acute upper airway obstruction the person most familiar with pediatric airway management should be called and arrangements made to quickly move the child to the operating room for endotracheal intubation under anesthesia. Traditionally, causative organisms include *Haemophilus influenzae* type b (Hib), *Streptococcus pneumoniae*, and group A streptococci. Secondary to the Hib vaccine the etiologic agents are changing.

Reference: Zitelli and Davis, pp. 721–2; Oski *et al.*, pp. 822–3

53. Answer: E

CPR always starts with airway, breathing, circulation and drugs. The child has a protected airway and is being ventilated and oxygenated with an ambu-bag. Chest compressions are being performed and cardiac medications are being administered via the endotracheal tube. There should be no delay in establishing intravenous access. If not obtained immediately there should be no hesitation in establishing intraosseous access in a pediatric patient. This is the preferred method of access prior to attempting a venous cutdown or a percutaneous central venous catheter.

Reference: Oski *et al.*, pp. 808–11

54. Answer: C

Carbon monoxide is the gas most commonly produced in a fire. Mild intoxication is a carboxyhemoglobin level of less than 20%, moderate 20–40%, and severe greater than 40%. Symptoms range from headache and dyspnea to shock, coma and hallucinations. Therapy is initiated with 100% oxygen and may include hyperbaric oxygen therapy. Initial evaluation includes a carboxyhemoglobin level, a complete blood count, arterial blood gas and chest radiograph.

Reference: Oski *et al.*, pp. 1489–90

55. Answer: D

G6PD deficiency is typically characterized by a low-grade, well tolerated hemolysis. Certain drugs and compounds, including fava beans, naphthalene (mothballs) and sulfa drugs, initiate an acute hemolysis that can result in jaundice and critical illness. G6PD deficiency is X-linked and over 370 variants have been isolated. Pyruvate kinase deficiency is usually a low-grade chronic hemolytic anemia not responsive to environmental triggers. Autoimmune hemolytic anemias usually take 3–7 days to present, not hours. Hereditary spherocytosis presents in the neonatal period. Paroxysmal nocturnal hemoglobinuria usually presents in late childhood and is characteristically worse during sleep and hemoglobinuria is present in the morning.

Reference: Zitelli and Davis, p. 320; Oski *et al.*, pp. 1663–6

56. Answer: E

This history and examination of this patient suggest a tension pneumothorax, which needs urgent decompression. This is best achieved immediately by passing a large gauge needle into the intrapleural space in the second intercostal space at the mid-clavicular line.

Reference: Sprigings *et al.*, p. 179

57. Answer: E

In an orbital blowout fracture, the affected site is the orbital floor with sparing of the orbital rim. There is a risk of prolapse of the orbital contents into the maxillary sinus with entrapment. Symptoms include pain, local tenderness, double vision (that disappears when one eye is covered), and eyelid swelling after nose blowing. One can have loss of sensation in the distribution of the infraorbital nerve (ipsilateral cheek and upper lip), tenderness as well as nosebleed. The use of nasal decongestants can minimize this. Surgical repair is an issue only if there is persistent double vision in the primary or reading position after several days when tissue swelling has lessened or if a large fracture is present. Double vision upon presentation is not an indication for emergent surgical intervention.

Reference: Wilson, pp. 364–5; Friedman *et al.*, pp. 2–4; Cullom and Chang, pp. 38–9

58. Answer: C

This patient is known to have symptoms consistent with peptic ulcer disease and now presents with severe nausea and vomiting. The physical examination points towards obstruction of the upper GI tract and in view of her history of peptic ulcer disease it is likely that there has been chronic scarring leading to gastric outlet obstruction.

Reference: Kelley, p. 612

59. Answer: A

The most likely metabolic imbalance in this patient is hypochloremic, hypokalemic metabolic alkalosis. Loss of hydrochloric acid from repeated vomiting leads to alkalosis and hypochloremia. The kidneys try to compensate for this by absorbing hydrogen in place of potassium leading to this metabolic upset.

Reference: Kelley, p. 978

60. Answer: A

Barriers to the initiation of ORT in industrialized countries generally come from the health care providers and their perceptions of ORT. These include: impracticalities of parental involvement in medical care, the time involved, the feeling that ORT can only be used in mild dehydration, and the fact that it cannot be used for vomiting children.

Reference: Oski *et al.*, pp. 856–8

61. Answer: C

Intussusception is the most common cause of intestinal obstruction in infants of 3–18 months of age. Intussusception occurs when a proximal portion of the bowel invaginates into a distal portion of the bowel. Any child with signs and symptoms of distal small bowel obstruction or colon obstruction, colicky pain or currant jelly stools (bloody mucus stools) should undergo a prompt diagnostic barium enema, that may be both diagnostic and therapeutic as it may reduce the invagination.

Reference: Zitelli and Davis, pp. 497–8; Oski et al., pp. 1856–8

62. Answer: E

Right lower quadrant pain in an adolescent or older female presents a sometimes difficult diagnosis, as there are a number of organs in that quadrant which may cause abdominal pain. Inflammatory bowel disease rarely presents with isolated abdominal pain symptoms, and usually has left lower quadrant pain.

Reference: Zitelli and Davis, p. 559; Oski et al., pp. 792, 1900–1

63. Answer: B

Flumazenil is a benzodiazepine receptor specific antagonist that has no effect on ethanol, barbiturates, or other sedative-hypnotic agents. It may induce seizures in patients with pre-existing seizure disorders, benzodiazepine addiction or concomitant tricyclic antidepressant overdose. If seizures occur, diazepam and other benzodiazepines will be less effective. As with naloxone, the duration of action of flumazenil is short and resedation might occur, requiring repeat doses.

Methylene blue enhances the conversion of methemoglobin to hemoglobin by increasing the activity of the enzyme hemoglobin reductase. Ethanol blocks metabolism of methanol and ethylene glycol by competing for the enzyme alcohol dehydrogenase. Naloxone is a specific opioid antagonist. It is structurally related to opioids but has no agonist effects. Acetylcysteine treatment is most effective if started within 8–10 hours of the overdose.

Reference: Tierney et al., pp. 1439–69

64. Answer: A

The history and examination are consistent with a diagnosis of pseudotumor cerebri. Chronic headache in an obese woman who has been treated with acne medication supports this diagnosis. A CT to exclude a space-occupying lesion followed by LP to measure CSF pressure should be done immediately. CSF pressure is typically raised and the ventricles on CT may be slit-like with periventricular lucencies. Visual acuity testing and visual field testing should be followed up by an ophthalmologist.

Reference: Samuels and Feske, pp. 1146–7

65. Answer: E

Acetazolamide is used in the treatment of pseudotumor cerebri. It is a carbonic anhydrase inhibitor, which reduces the formation of CSF. Other treatments include steroids and diuretics. Lumbar–peritoneal shunting may also be helpful in difficult cases. All the other agents, especially tetracyclines and acne medications containing vitamin A or its derivatives, can precipitate pseudotumor cerebri.

Reference: Samuels and Feske, pp. 1146–7

66. Answer: C

This patient is severely hemodynamically compromised. DC cardioversion at 100 J is the best option. Verapamil and adenosine have a role in the treatment of the stable patient with supraventricular tachycardia after vagal maneuvers. In some instances, providing cardioversion is not delayed, a short trial of adenosine may be tried while the patient is being prepared for cardioversion.

Reference: Cummins, pp. 1.33, 1.34

67. Answer: D

Corneal, gag, oculocephalic and pupillary reflexes are all brain stem reflexes and will be absent in brain death. Ankle jerks and other peripheral reflexes can still be present as these are spinal reflexes and do not require the brain stem. Decerebrate and decorticate posturing require an intact brain stem and therefore are incompatible with brain stem death.

68. Answer: C

The strip in Figure 6 shows atrial fibrillation. Note the irregular R–R interval and that no P waves are seen. The QRS complex is normal in size and duration and is followed by a normal T wave.

Reference: Cummins, p. 3.11

69. Answer: D

All the drugs listed except for adenosine are useful in the treatment of atrial fibrillation. Digoxin can be used for rate control but takes many hours to work and is not suitable when immediate rate control is required. Digoxin will not cardiovert the patient back into sinus rhythm. Rate control with a short-acting β-blocker or a calcium channel blocker may also be considered. Amiodarone and procainamide are useful for rate control and cardioversion. Another option is electrical cardioversion. It is important to note that atrial fibrillation and atrial flutter increase the risk of cardio-embolic events and anticoagulation with heparin and warfarin reduces this risk. In general, if atrial fibrillation is present for longer than 48 hours, anticoagulation for 1 month pre- and post-cardioversion is recommended. Adenosine is helpful in the management of supraventricular tachycardia but has no role in atrial fibrillation.

Reference: Cummins, pp. 3.11, 4.6

70. Answer: D

This is Mobitz 2:1 block (Figure 7). Note that not all P waves are followed by a QRS complex. It is not important in itself but may precede complete heart block.

Reference: Hampton, p. 264

71. Answer: E

Several large cooperative studies, most notably the Coronary Artery Surgery Study (CASS), have examined outcomes for patients with coronary artery disease treated with medical vs. surgical intervention. The following are considered formal indications for CABG, and medical professionals working with patients suffering from coronary artery disease should be highly familiar with them:

Anatomical disease:

Significant left main coronary artery disease
Double or triple vessel disease involving proximal LAD

Symptomatic disease:

Unstable angina
Post-MI angina
Acute coronary occlusion after PTCA
Angina unsuccessfully controlled with medical therapy
Unacceptable lifestyle with medical therapy

Reference: Greenfield, p. 1543

72. Answer: D

Delirium is a disturbance of consciousness, accompanied by a change in cognition that cannot be accounted for by pre-existing dementia. The disturbance is acute, developing in hours or days, and has a fluctuating course. There is reduced awareness of the environment, and impaired ability to focus, sustain or shift attention. These patients also have memory or language disturbances and disorientation, and perceptual illusions and hallucinations are common. Delirium is also often associated with a disturbance in the sleep–wake cycle, and the individual may exhibit anxiety, fear, irritability, anger, depression, euphoria or apathy. Physical examination and laboratories provide an etiological explanation, or the history is consistent with intoxication or withdrawal of psychoactive substances.

Reference: DSM–IV, pp. 124–5

73. Answer: B

The essential feature of body dysmorphic disorder is a pre-occupation with an imagined defect in appearance which causes significant distress or impairment in social, occupational or other important areas of functioning. If a slight physical anomaly is present, the individual's concern is markedly excessive. Complaints most commonly involve the face or head, but any other body part may be involved. Frequent checking of the perceived flaw, with attendant severe anxiety, is very common. Excessive grooming and attempts at camouflaging the 'defect' are common, as are often requests for reassurance which, however, provide only temporary relief. Avoidance can lead to severe isolation, work impairment and family difficulties. The distress and dysfunction associated with the disease can lead to hospitalizations, suicidal ideation, suicide attempts and completed suicide. Individuals with this disorder often pursue medical, dental or surgical treatment to rectify their imagined defect. Such treatment may cause worsening of the disorder, leading to repeated interventions.

Reference: DSM–IV, pp. 466–7

74. Answer: C

This patient most probably has mucormycosis, a life-threatening fungal infection occurring in poorly controlled diabetics and immunocompromised patients. *Rhizopus* and *Rhizomucor* are ubiquitous and appear on decaying vegetation, dung and foods of high sugar content. Mucormycosis can occur in the sinuses, lung and gastrointestinal tract. Vascular invasion by hyphae is a prominent feature. Ischemic or hemorrhagic necrosis is the foremost histologic finding. The organism is difficult to grow from infected tissue. Treatment consists of good control of the diabetes mellitus or decrease in immunosuppressive drugs, extensive surgical debridement and amphotericin B. Azoles are of no value. Mortality from the disease is high.

Reference: Fauci *et al.*, p. 1158

75. Answer: D

HIVAN has a striking predilection for African-American individuals. HIVAN is 7–10 times more common in men than in women and 30–60% have a history of intravenous drug abuse. Clinical manifestations are heavy proteinuria, azotemia, normal blood pressure, enlarged kidneys and rapid progression to end-stage renal disease. Antiretroviral treatment appears to delay progression.

Reference: Greenberg *et al.*, p. 239

76. Answer: C

Acute MI, bleeding from anastomotic sites, infection and aortoenteric fistula are the most common severe complications of AAA repair. Infection is a rare (1%) but particularly serious complication and mandates the removal of infected material and an extra-anatomic approach to restoring distal blood flow. The diagnosis of infected graft material is usually made in a patient with recent placement of graft material that is persistently febrile with positive blood cultures. Replacing an infected graft with new uninfected material generally does not allow for a sufficient margin of uninfected vasculature proximally and/or distally and is not performed. Aorto-aortic bypass is not attempted for a similar reason. Medical therapy is almost uniformly futile. Axillobifemoral bypass is the procedure of choice, accompanied by occlusion of the aorta. A distal point of bifurcation is superior to a proximal bifurcation as it allows for a higher rate of flow across the main portion of the bypass graft.

Reference: Sabiston, p. 1671

77. Answer: D

This patient is in oliguric renal failure, defined as a urine output of less than 400 ml/day. His recent sepsis and prolonged hypovolemia are likely etiologic agents. Endotoxins, notably lipid A from the cell walls of gram-negative organisms, have been implicated as a contributing cause to multiple organ system failure in sepsis. While acute tubular necrosis (ATN) is actually a histologic diagnosis, examination of this patient gives several important reasons to infer a presumptive diagnosis: rapid loss of renal function, rising BUN and absence of extrarenal or prerenal causes. Much work has been done on the pathophysiology of the initiation and maintenance of ATN and acute renal failure (ARF). The likely etiologic factor in this patient's renal dysfunction is ischemia, with constriction of the afferent arterioles in the nephric circulation. Ischemic insult leads to a variety of functional impairments. Back-leakage across injured tubular epithelium and increased intratubular back-pressures have been implicated in the pathophysiology of tubular injury. There is a resultant increase in the concentration of many circulating toxins. Urea is by itself not a clinically significant toxin, but serves as an effective surrogate marker for the accumulation of toxic compounds that are more difficult to assay.

Reference: Sabiston, p. 363

78. Answer: C

Superior mesenteric artery (SMA) syndrome is a relatively rare cause of gastrointestinal obstruction, but it is associated with dramatic weight loss, scoliosis, supine immobilization and circumferential body casts. In this syndrome, the SMA either partially or completely obstructs the distal third portion of the duodenum. Persistent nausea, vomiting, and distention are classic clinical features. The mesenteric fat helps to buoy the small intestine and transverse colon (and subsequently the SMA) away from the duodenum, and in patients with weight loss, it is believed the loss of this fat leads to duodenal obstruction. The best test to demonstrate the point of obstruction is an upper GI series. CT scan and fluoroscopy are also helpful in making the radiologic diagnosis. Angiography may be helpful in conjunction with an upper GI series but not as a primary study. Other syndromes can present in a similar fashion, but the workup would still involve a study to delineate the functional anatomy of the upper GI tract.

Reference: Sabiston, pp. 888–9

79. Answer: C

Esophageal atresia and TEF are a relatively common congenital defect, occurring in 1 : 1500–1 : 3000 live births. There is no greater incidence in either sex. The condition is associated with several genetic syndromes, including trisomy 18 (Edward syndrome), trisomy 21 (Down syndrome), and VACTERL (vertebral, anal, cardiac, tracheoesophageal, renal and limb abnormalities) syndrome. There are five major variants of TEF, the most commonly encountered being type C (85%) as described in option A in the question. The most common long-term complications after repair of TEF include reflux, stricture, tracheomalacia and leak. An anti-reflux procedure is commonly required to control symptoms.

Reference: Sabiston, p. 1237

80. Answer: A

Dobutamine is a synthetic sympathomimetic amine. It acts on both β-1 and α-adrenergic receptors causing an increase in cardiac output. The β-effect outbalances the α-effect causing vasodilation and increases coronary blood flow. Higher doses produce tachycardia and should be avoided.

Reference: Cummins, p. 8.5

81. Answer: C

Norepinephrine has both β-1 and α-adrenergic effects but only little β-2. The result is marked vasoconstriction and a positive inotropic effect on the heart. It should be used as a last resort in patients with coronary artery disease as it can exacerbate myocardial ischemia. Extravasation of norepinephrine at the infusion site can cause severe necrosis; infusion of the affected area with phentolamine can reduce this severe effect.

Reference: Cummins, p. 8.3

82. Answer: C

There is enough information to help us make the diagnosis of Wegener granulomatosis. This woman has sinusitis, renal failure, hematuria and pulmonary involvement causing hemoptysis. In addition she has mononeuritis multiplex. The other conditions, especially Goodpasture syndrome, can give one or more of the findings but sinusitis, renal and pulmonary involvement would best fit with Wegener granulomatosis. Sinusitis is not typically associated with Goodpasture syndrome.

Reference: Kelley, p.1165

83. Answer: B

cANCA are present in over 95% of active cases of Wegener granulomatosis. pANCA is positive in 50% of polyarteritis nodosa cases, 70% of Churg–Strauss and 70% of idiopathic crescentic glomerulonephritis and 20% of Wegener syndrome. Anti-GBM antibodies are positive in over 90% of Goodpasture cases and antimitochondrial antibodies are positive in over 90% of primary biliary cirrhosis patients.

Reference: Kelley, pp. 1164–5, 2043–4

84.   Answer: A

Only lidocaine, epinephrine and atropine can be administered through the endotracheal tube.

Reference: Cummins, p. 2.3

85.   Answer: C

This girl has developed an acute dystonic reaction from administration of an anti-emetic agent. Acute dystonia or oculogyric crisis are well recognized side-effects of dopamine antagonist anti-emetic agents. Intramuscular benztropine, or another anticholinergic agent, is the immediate appropriate action.

Reference: Samuels and Feske, p. 666

86.   Answer: A

The history of malaise, nausea, vomiting, dark mucus membranes, dark palmar creases, and now hyperkalemia, hyponatremia and hypotension would make adrenocortical deficiency the likely diagnosis. The patient currently is in adrenocortical crisis which is a medical emergency. The cause of the adrenal insufficiency is unclear and may be primary or secondary. There is no evidence to support the other given diagnoses.

Reference: Kelley, pp. 2219–20

87.   Answer: B

The immediate course of action is hospitalization. Fluid replacement should begin aggressively with saline and a glucocorticoid should also be given. Treatment should not be delayed for diagnostic testing. However, if dexamethasone is given instead of hydrocortisone then cosyntropin testing can begin as treatment is taking place. Cosyntropin is a synthetic ACTH. Plasma cortisol is measured before and after administration of cosyntropin.

Reference: Kelley, pp. 2220–1

88.   Answer: C

Appropriate tests include biopsy to look for histological evidence of non-caseating granuloma, chest X-ray to look for lung involvement and bilateral hilar lymphadenopathy. The serum angiotensin-converting enzyme is of limited value in the initial diagnosis as it is elevated in only two-thirds of patients but can be used to follow the course of the disease. The Kveim test is no longer available in most centers and involves intradermal injection of sarcoid spleen tissue. If positive, non-caseating granulomas are seen at the site of injection after 4–6 weeks.

Reference: Kelley, p. 2019

89.   Answer: E

Hypopituitarism, seizures and peripheral neuropathy are some of the features of neurosarcoid. Dyspnea is a common complaint owing to pulmonary involvement. Sarcoid can affect many organs, giving a wide range of symptoms. There is no proven link between sarcoidosis and inflammatory bowel disease.

Reference: Kelley, p. 2019

90.   Answer: D

Cholelithiasis, cataract formation, and delayed hemorrhage are the three most common delayed complications after electrical burn injury. Cholelithiasis and cataracts have been reported up to 3 years after the initial injury. Delayed hemorrhage can occur, often from blood vessels of significant caliber, usually within the few weeks after an injury. More immediate complications include visceral injury (pancreas, liver, intestine, pancreatic necrosis, gallbladder injury), as well as a range of neurologic injuries. Pituitary dysfunction is not a commonly reported complication.

Reference: Sabiston, p. 238

91.   Answer: B

This woman has developed a retroperitoneal hemorrhage while on anticoagulants. The absence of the right knee reflex and iliopsoas weakness suggests L2–L4 involvement. The history is inconsistent with GBS and ruptured aortic aneurysm. A pelvic tumor is a possibility and a CT of the abdomen and pelvis is required to exclude this.

Reference: Bradley et al., pp. 2040–1

92.   Answer: D

Protamine sulfate will reverse the effect of heparin at a dose of 1mg per 100 units given. Vitamin K antagonizes the anticoagulant effect of warfarin. Desferrioxamine is used in the treatment of hemochromatosis. Factor VIII replacement is given to hemophiliacs to correct the coagulopathy.

Reference: Kelley, p. 572

93.   Answer: C

Ten to 15 per cent of stones are composed of magnesium and ammonium phosphate (struvite or infection stones). Struvite stones are formed in the presence of a high concentration of ammonia in urine having persistently alkaline pH (greater than 7.5). Under normal circumstances alkaline urine has a low concentration of ammonia. In patients with urinary tract infections caused by urea-splitting organisms, especially *Proteus* species, the bacterial urease hydrolyzes urea to form ammonia and bicarbonate. The resulting urine has an alkaline pH and is supersaturated with calcium phosphate. The high ammonia concentration in urine leads to the formation of magnesium and ammonium phosphate crystals, which aggregate and become stones. Hypercalciuria, and a small volume of very concentrated urine, can also contribute to the pathogenesis of struvite stones. Uric acid and cysteine stone formation is enhanced by an increased urinary acidity.

Reference: Dornbrand *et al.*, pp. 274–81

94. Answer: A

Age is not a contraindication for thrombolysis; however, prognosis after MI is worse in the elderly. Absolute contra-indications are active bleeding, defective hemostasis, recent major trauma, surgical procedures less than 10 days prior to infarction, neurosurgical procedures within the last 2 months, prolonged CPR (longer than 10 minutes), history of stroke in the last year, cerebral tumor, aneurysm or AVM, acute pericarditis, suspected aortic dissection, active peptic ulcer disease, active cavitating lung disease and pregnancy.

Reference: Ewald and McKenzie, p. 99

95. Answer: E

Invasive otitis externa is a potentially life-threatening infection that slowly invades from the external canal into adjacent soft tissues, mastoid, and temporal bones and eventually spreads across the base of the skull. It occurs primarily in diabetic patients whose diabetes is under control. In more than 95% of cases *Pseudomonas aeruginosa* is the pathogen involved; in the remaining cases the pathogens include *Staphylococcus epidermidis*, *Aspergillus*, *Fusobacterium* and *Actinomyces*.

Reference: Fauci *et al.*, p.181

96. Answer: C

Confounding occurs whenever there is a mixing of the effect of the exposure and the disease with a third factor that itself is associated with the exposure and is independently associated with the disease. Because there is an association between smoking and alcohol use, and because alcohol use has already been shown to have an effect on psoriasis, this study could be marred by the presence of confounding.

Reference: Hennekens *et al.*, 287–323

97. Answer: B

Since mothers of children with birth defects are more likely to recall every possible event that may have contributed to their children's problems, the issue of recall bias is a major concern here. Again, other biases and issues such as con-founding are certainly important, but they are less likely to play as major a role in this study.

Reference: Hennekens *et al.*, pp. 272–86

98. Answer: E

The data in this text were apparently derived from a cross-sectional study which essentially represented a snapshot in time regarding how many women had carcinoma. The population used in this text, however, may not reflect your patient, since she may have different risk factors for acquiring the disease. Therefore, such prevalence estimates provide only a rough idea of how likely this patient is to have cancer. Because we are examining prevalence data rather than incidence data, this would include women who have preva-lent cancer but acquired it prior to age 40. Finally, because these data are cross-sectional, women who acquired cancer but died quickly before the study was undertaken would not be reflected in the study. These are some of the issues that make the use of cross-sectional studies, and prevalence studies in particular, problematic.

Reference: Hennekens *et al.*, pp. 54–98

99. Answer: B

The only possible answer from the list is B. The others are all statistical tests that are not used to estimate survival. The Kaplan–Meier product limit estimator is a useful and straightforward way to estimate the absolute probability of survival at a given point in time in the presence of censoring. (Censored observations refer to patients who do not reach the disease endpoint during their period of follow-up.)

Reference: Rosner, pp. 607–9

These color illustrations refer to the correspondingly numbered questions in Test Four (page 91).

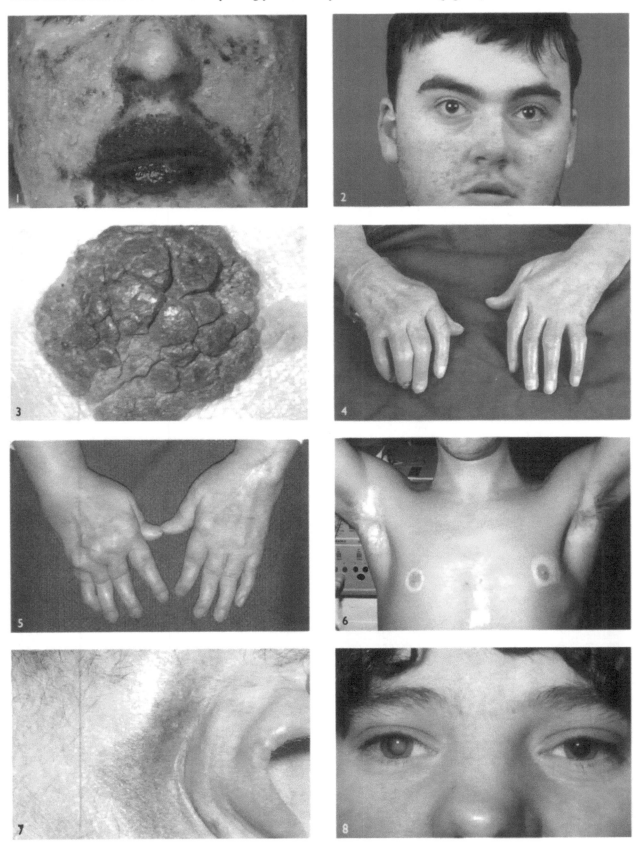

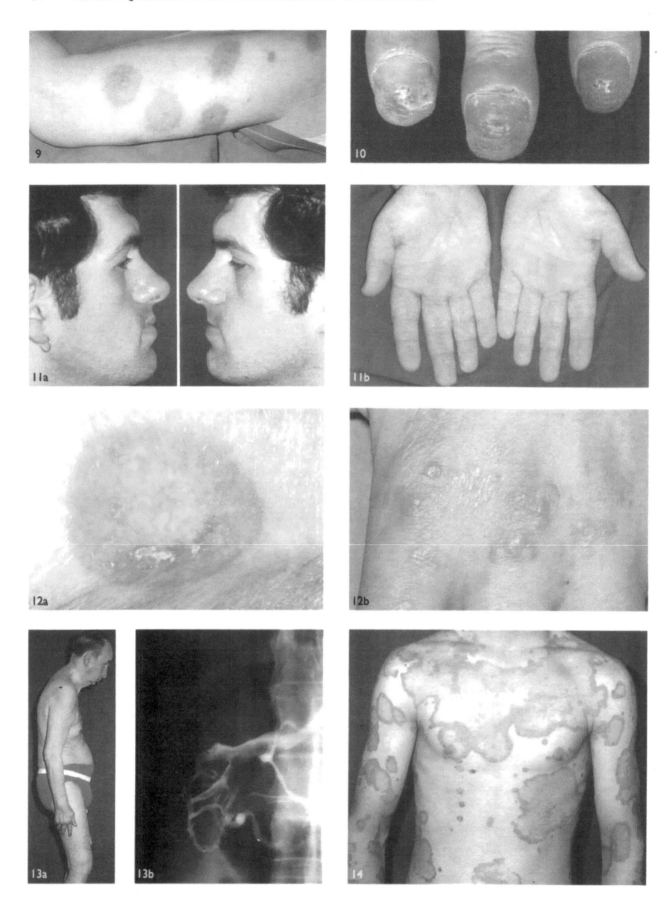

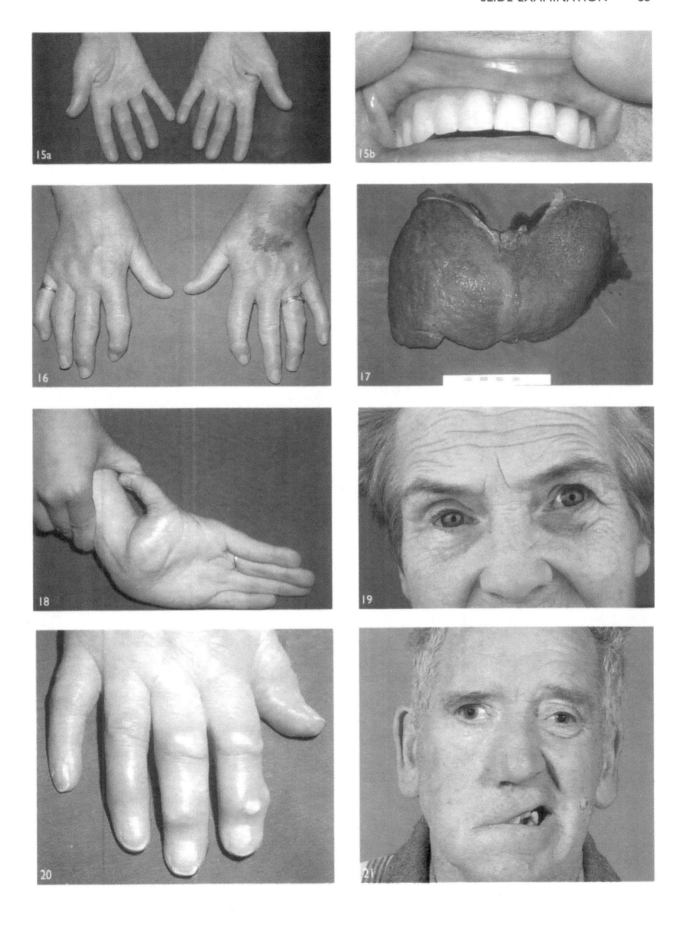

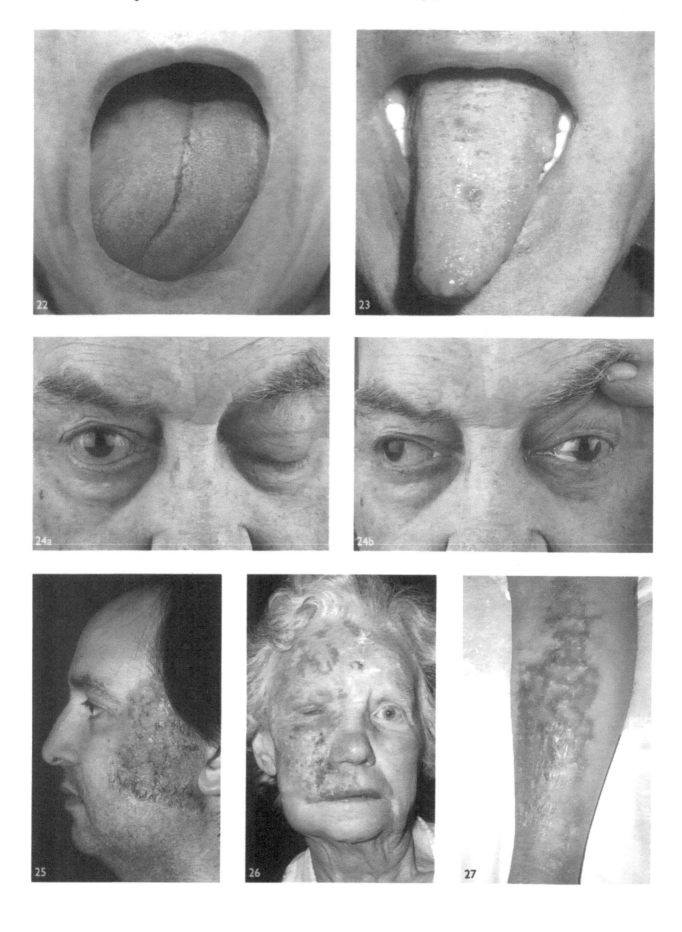

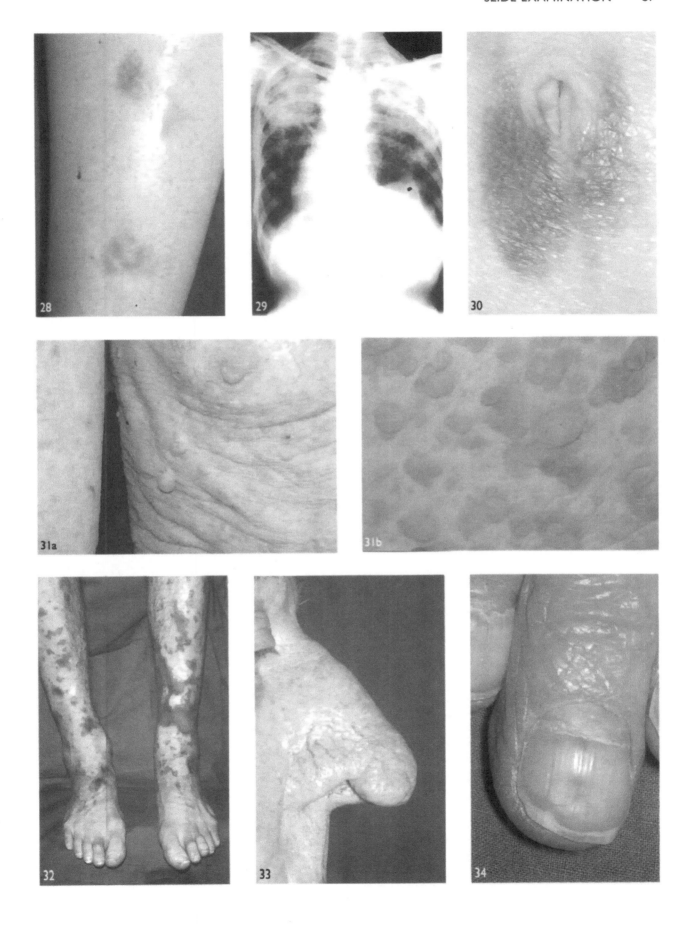

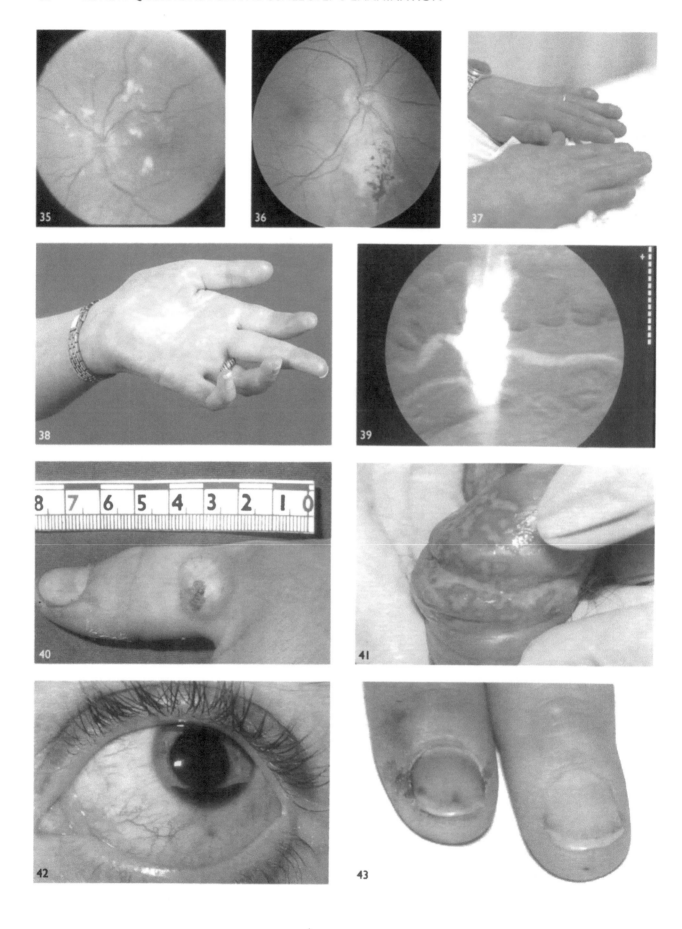

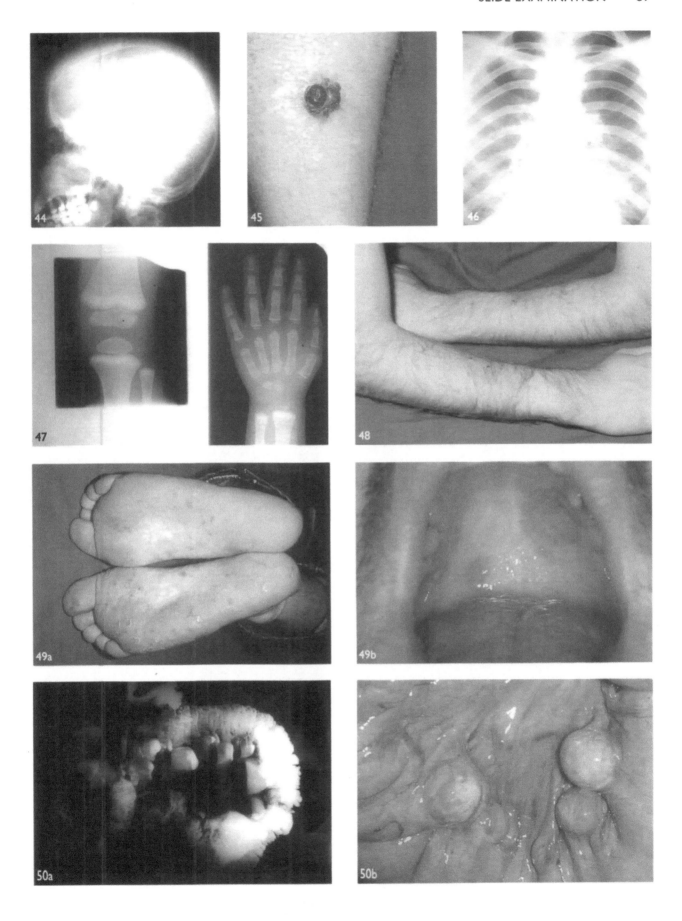

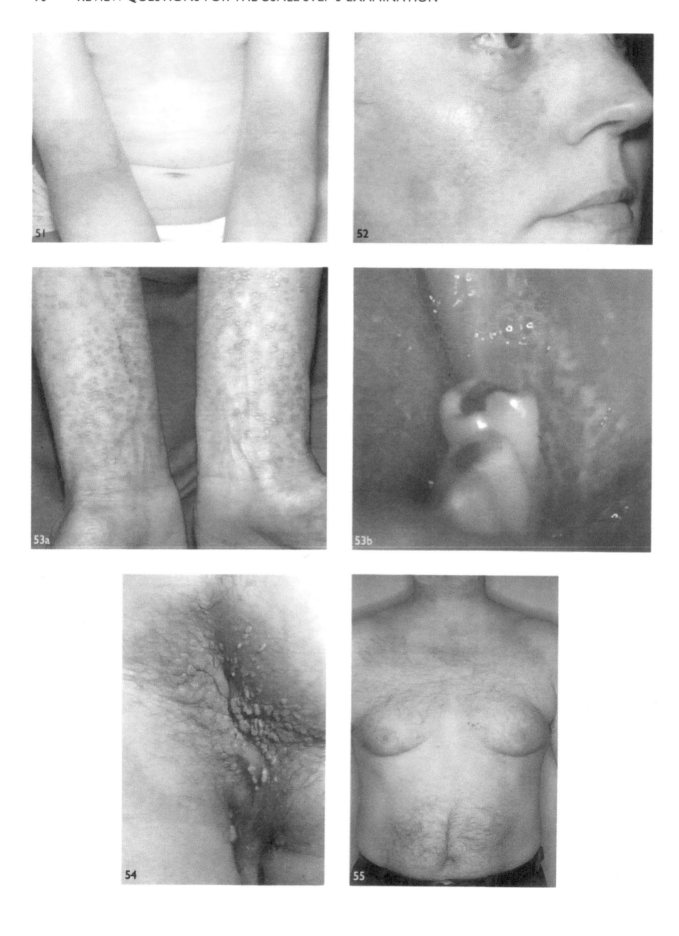

TEST FOUR

Slide examination

For questions 1–55 refer to the correspondingly numbered color slide or slides.

1. A 23-year-old woman presented to the ER with the facial appearance shown. The day prior to this presentation, she was prescribed an antibiotic for a chest infection by her primary care physician. She has target lesions all over her body.

This appearance is consistent with:

A. pemphigoid
B. labial herpes simplex infection
C. angioneurotic edema
D. severe psoriasis
E. Stevens–Johnson syndrome

2. This 15-year-old boy is mentally retarded and has epilepsy. The likely diagnosis is:

A. tuberous sclerosis
B. Down syndrome
C. acne vulgaris
D. acne rosacea
E. Klinefelter syndrome

3. A 73-year-old man comes to your office with a 10-year history of this lesion on his back. The lesion is:

A. basal cell papilloma
B. malignant melanoma
C. rodent ulcer
D. pigmented hairy nevus
E. metastases

4A. The hands of a 55-year-old woman are shown. What is the likely diagnosis?

A. rheumatoid arthritis
B. scleroderma
C. lupus
D. osteoarthritis
E. sarcoid

4B. Known complications of scleroderma include all the following except:

A. heart failure
B. malabsorption
C. dysphagia
D. dyspnea
E. infertility

5. These are the hands of a 65-year-old woman. What is the likely diagnosis?

A. osteoarthritis
B. gout
C. rheumatoid arthritis
D. scleroderma
E. sarcoid

6A. This 24-year-old Indian man comes to the office with these lesions. The affected areas have normal sensation. Examination is otherwise normal. The likely diagnosis is:

A. leprosy
B. vitiligo
C. psoriasis
D. lichen planus

6B. All of the following are associated with the condition shown in slide 6 except:

A. diabetes mellitus type II
B. pernicious anemia
C. thyroid disease
D. Addison disease
E. renal failure

7. This man was involved in a motor vehicle accident. This sign is called:

A. Battle's sign
B. Cullen's sign
C. Murphy's sign
D. Trouseau's sign
E. Tinel's sign

8. This woman has noticed decreased vision in the right eye. Causes of this lesion include all of the following except:

A. steroids
B. aging
C. exposure to radiation
D. digoxin
E. chronic irritation of the eye

9A. A 39-year-old male comes to the office with this lesion. All of the following are potential causes of this lesion except:

A. ulcerative colitis
B. Crohn disease
C. rheumatoid arthritis
D. dysproteinemia
E. Lyme disease

9B. On further questioning he admits to diarrhea and blood in his stools most mornings and intermittent abdominal pain. Appropriate investigations include all of the following except:

A. CBC and electrolytes
B. barium meal and gastroscopy
C. colonoscopy
D. stools cultures and microscopy
E. erythrocyte sedimentation rate (ESR)

10.   What condition is associated with these nail changes?

A. psoriasis
B. lupus
C. fungal infection
D. gout

11.   This 24-year-old tall male comes to your office because of difficulty with his vision at work. He attributes two accidents at work to his poor vision. He also complains of paresthesia of his hands and generalized weakness. In addition, he is impotent. On examination, his blood pressure is elevated at 170/105. He has very prominent facial features and large hands and feet. All the following are useful in the initial investigations except:

A. old photographs of the patient
B. oral glucose tolerance test
C. CT scan of the brain
D. visual field testing
E. visual evoked potentials

12.   A 52-year-old woman comes to your office with this lesion on her arm. What is it?

A. granuloma annulare
B. necrobiosis lipoidica
C. psoriasis
D. pretibial myxedema

13A. The patient shown undergoes a renal arteriogram and venogram. The venogram shown shows renal vein thrombosis. What is the likely diagnosis from the appearance of the patient and the vertebral spine?

A. ankylosing spondylitis
B. rheumatoid arthritis
C. osteoporosis
D. osteomyelitis

13B. Clinical features of ankylosing spondylitis include all the following except:

A. apical pulmonary fibrosis
B. plantar tendinitis
C. sacroiliitis
D. back pain
E. renal artery and vein thrombosis

14A. A 25-year-old woman comes to your office with the skin lesion shown. The diagnosis is:

A. psoriasis
B. meningococcal septicemia
C. pityriasis rosea
D. Henoch–Schönlein purpura

14B. All the following drugs aggravate this condition except:

A. β-blockers
B. lithium
C. chloroquine
D. steroids

15.   This man was seen in the ER with hypotension, hyperkalemia and hyponatremia. What is the likely diagnosis?

A. Cushing disease
B. Addison disease
C. lichen planus
D. anemia

16.   What is the most likely cause of the appearance of this patient's hands:

A. rheumatoid arthritis
B. osteoarthritis
C. lupus
D. sarcoid
E. scleroderma

17.   All of the following can cause changes in the liver that are shown, except:

A. alcohol
B. primary biliary cirrhosis
C. diabetes
D. Wilson disease
E. hemachromatosis

18.   What is the likely diagnosis?

A. Ehlers–Danlos syndrome
B. pseudoxanthoma elasticum
C. Marfan syndrome
D. acromegaly

19. The woman shown in slide 19 had an upper respiratory tract infection and was constantly coughing. She comes to the ER complaining of right-sided neck pain and weakness and numbness of her left arm. She also noticed a 'difference between the two sides of her face'. The history and facial appearance could be consistent with:

A. right carotid dissection
B. left carotid dissection
C. basilar artery thrombosis
D. compression fractures of the cervical vertebrae
E. left middle cerebral artery stroke

20. What is the cause of the appearance of this patient's hand?

A. chronic tophaceous gout
B. osteoarthritis
C. sarcoid
D. rheumatoid arthritis

21. This patient has been asked to smile. What cranial nerve is affected?

A. oculomotor
B. facial
C. abducens
D. glossopharyngeal
E. olfactory

22. This patient was asked to stick her tongue out. Which cranial nerve is affected?

A. left hypoglossal
B. right hypoglossal
C. left trigeminal
D. right trigeminal
E. vagus

23. This woman has recurrent GI bleeding. What is the likely diagnosis?

A. Rendu–Osler–Weber syndrome
B. neurofibromatosis
C. Hermansky–Pudlak syndrome
D. pseudoxanthoma elasticum
E. Ehlers–Danlos syndrome

24. This 65-year-old male presents to the ER because of blurred vision and droopy eyelid. Which cranial nerve is affected?

A. oculomotor
B. trochlear
C. abducens
D. trigeminal
E. facial

25. A 35-year-old man comes to the clinic with these lesions. Lateral pressure of the skin appeared to cause the epidermis to slide over the dermis. What is the diagnosis?

A. bullous pemphigoid
B. dermatitis herpetiformis
C. pemphigus vulgaris
D. drug reaction

26. This homeless woman presents to the ER with this lesion. The likely diagnosis is:

A. herpes simplex
B. molluscum contagiosum
C. pyoderma gangrenosum
D. butterfly rash of lupus
E. herpes zoster

27. This 85-year-old woman with a history of hypo-thyroidism came to the clinic with this lesion. The likely diagnosis is:

A. erythema ab igne
B. deep venous thrombosis
C. pretibial myxedema
D. necrobiosis lipoidica
E. granuloma annulare

28. This 33-year-old woman has a peripheral neuropathy and cataracts. She also complains of pruritus vulvae. The likely diagnosis is:

A. diabetes mellitus
B. hypothyroidism
C. hyperthyroidism
D. hypoparathyroidism

29. This chest X-ray is from a 28-year-old man who presents with cough, weight loss, cervical lymphadenopathy and night sweats. The likely diagnosis is:

A. pulmonary fibrosis
B. pleural thickening
C. metastatic carcinoma
D. coarctation of the aorta
E. TB

30. This patient, who had a history of excess alcohol, is seen in the ER with sudden-onset abdominal pain. He is hemodynamically stable and all the peripheral pulses are palpable. What is the likely diagnosis?

A. perforated diverticulum
B. perforated ulcer
C. acute pancreatitis
D. acute cholecystitis
E. dissected aortic aneurysm

31. Which one of the following is not associated with this condition?

A. hypertension
B. multiple endocrine neoplasia
C. peripheral nerve lesions
D. hearing problems
E. X-linked inheritance

32. This patient presented to the ER with fever, photophobia and neck stiffness. The most likely diagnosis is:

A. viral meningitis
B. Stevens–Johnson syndrome
C. drug reaction
D. Henoch–Schönlein purpura
E. meningococcal meningitis

33. A concerned daughter brings her elderly father to your office. She tells you that his nose is getting 'redder and bigger'. What is the diagnosis?

A. rhinophyma
B. lupus pernio
C. acne vulgaris
D. basal cell carcinoma

34. A 35-year-old woman comes to your office with the nail changes shown. She was recently discharged from the local hospital for septicemia following a motor vehicle accident. These nail changes are associated with which of the following:

A. fungal infection of the nails
B. nail-patella syndrome
C. convalescence from serious systemic illness
D. wrist drop

35. This is the fundus of a patient with headaches and confusion. His blood pressure is 180/133. His chest X-ray shows mild pulmonary edema. The likely diagnosis is:

A. diabetic retinopathy
B. retinitis pigmentosa
C. grade IV hypertensive retinopathy
D. grade I hypertensive retinopathy

36. You are examining the fundus of a 5-year-old girl who has just immigrated to the United States from South America. The likely diagnosis is:

A. retinitis pigmentosa
B. diabetic retinopathy
C. hypertensive retinopathy
D. drusen
E. glaucoma

37. This gentleman comes to the clinic concerned about the appearance of his fingers. All the following are recognized causes of clubbing except:

A. lung tumor
B. inflammatory bowel disease
C. chronic obstructive pulmonary disease (COPD)
D. bacterial endocarditis
E. pulmonary fibrosis

38. This 22-year-old patient comes to your office. A lesion of which nerve has caused this appearance of the hand:

A. ulnar
B. median
C. lateral cutaneous nerve
D. radial nerve

39. This is an angiogram of a 56-year-old man. All of the following statements about this patient are true except:

A. angiotensin-converting enzyme inhibitors can be used without concern in this patient
B. this patient is likely to be hypertensive and blood pressure control will be difficult
C. this patient is at risk for coronary artery disease
D. this patient is likely to have retinopathy

40. A veterinary student working on a sheep farm comes to your office with this lesion. What is it?

A. molluscum contagiosum
B. herpes simplex
C. common wart
D. orf
E. herpes zoster

41. This 25-year-old man developed these penile lesions. What is the diagnosis?

A. syphilitic chancre
B. genital herpes
C. fungal infection
D. chlamydia

42. A 25-year-old man is concerned about the appearance of his eye. The likely diagnosis is:

A. trauma to the eye
B. diabetes
C. hypertension
D. lupus
E. sarcoid

43. This 24-year-old woman developed shortness of breath, fever and these lesions. Two days earlier she had gone to the dentist for a routine check-up. You suspect bacterial endocarditis. All of the following clinical signs would help to support your diagnosis except:

A. splenomegaly
B. hematuria
C. heart murmur
D. retinal vasculitis
E. macroglossia

44. This is the X-ray of the skull of a 5-year-old Burmese boy who recently arrived in the USA. What is the diagnosis?

A. thalassemia
B. acute myeloid leukemia
C. lead poisoning
D. fracture of the skull

45. A 25-year-old farmer comes to your office with this lesion. What is the diagnosis?

A. melanoma
B. birth mark
C. basal cell papilloma
D. basal cell carcinoma
E. pigmented nevus

46. This is the chest X-ray of a patient with HIV infection. What is the likely diagnosis?

A. *Pneumocystis carinii* pneumonia
B. metastatic lung disease
C. pulmonary fibrosis
D. bronchiectasis

47. Which one of these blood tests would be most helpful in establishing the diagnosis for this child, who presents with increasing weakness and somnolence?

A. liver function tests
B. thyroid function
C. blood smear
D. serum lead
E. serum calcium

48. All the drugs listed below can cause this appearance except:

A. cyclosporine
B. steroids
C. phenytoin
D. amiodarone
E. minoxidil

49. A 35-year-old man presents with joint pain, pustular lesions on the soles of his feet and painless ulcers of his mouth. He also complains of a red eye. Ten days earlier he had severe diarrhea. What is the likely diagnosis?

A. pustular psoriasis
B. Reiter syndrome
C. rheumatoid arthritis
D. osteoarthritis

50. A 67-year-old man was killed in a road traffic accident. The incidental finding at autopsy is shown. His medical records show that he underwent a barium study 2 weeks earlier for weight loss. The likely diagnosis is:

A. colonic diverticulosis
B. ulcerative colitis
C. Crohn disease
D. small bowel diverticulosis
E. colonic carcinoma

51. A 15-year-old has itchy areas of skin and occasional difficulty with breathing at night. All the following are associated with this condition except:

A. asthma
B. hay fever
C. food intolerance and allergy
D. molluscum contagiosum
E. diabetes

52. A 22-year-old woman comes to your office concerned about the rash on her face. She also complains of joint pains. Which condition is this rash characteristic of?

A. lupus
B. sarcoid
C. scleroderma
D. atopic eczema
E. psoriasis

53. This woman developed these severely itchy lesions after starting a diuretic for heart failure. The likely lesion is:

A. psoriasis
B. lichen planus
C. lichen sclerosis
D. molluscum contagiosum

54. This 35-year-old man comes to the clinic with these lesions. All the following statements are correct about this condition except:

A. these lesions are not infective
B. they are caused by human papilloma virus
C. they spontaneously regress over months and years
D. the commonest site for men is the penis
E. the commonest site in women is the introitus

55. A 45-year-old man comes to your office for an annual check-up. You notice the changes shown in the photograph. Which of the following is not associated with this condition?

A. cimetidine
B. liver disease
C. testicular tumors
D. digoxin
E. ranitidine

Other encounters

56. Which of the following statements is FALSE concerning omphalocele and gastroschisis?

A. omphalocele is midline, whereas gastroschisis usually occurs to the right of midline
B. both omphalocele and gastroschisis are associated with elevated maternal levels of AFP
C. omphalocele generally has no sac enclosing the herniation, whereas gastroschisis usually does
D. treatment of omphalocele is generally less emergent than treatment of gastroschisis

57. Your patient is a 23-year-old woman who has suffered a closed head injury in a motor vehicle crash and is now in a persistent vegetative state. She has signed an organ donor card and her family respects her wishes regarding the use of her organs. Which of the following is TRUE about the procurement and transplantation of her liver?

A. patients with primary cholestatic disease have the best outcomes after liver transplantation
B. her liver will not be transplanted into a patient with cirrhosis due to alcoholism because of the likelihood of recidivism
C. the liver has the shortest allowable preservation time of any of the transplantable organs
D. partial transplantation, usually with the right lobe of the liver, is the procedure of choice for children with biliary atresia
E. none of the above is true

58. The liver from the donor patient in question 57 is transplanted into a 35-year-old woman suffering from primary biliary cirrhosis (PBC). Which of the following is TRUE regarding the physiology of the transplanted liver, and the complications that can arise in the postoperative period?

A. primary nonfunction can occur up to 1 week after transplantation
B. portal vein thrombosis is a common complication
C. most cases of hepatic artery thrombosis are due to technical flaws
D. the sole blood supply of the common bile duct is the hepatic artery

59. The following are risk factors for breast cancer except:

A. early menopause
B. early menarche
C. family history of breast carcinoma
D. late first pregnancy

60. The following statements regarding venous thrombosis are correct except:

A. emboli are more likely to originate in calf veins than thigh veins
B. clinical diagnosis is often difficult and unreliable
C. venograms are helpful in the diagnosis
D. labeled fibrinogen scanning can help in the diagnosis

61. Alcohol intoxication-related sleep disturbances include all the following except:

A. suppression of REM sleep in the first half of the night
B. multiple awakenings in the second half of the night
C. episodic sleep apnea
D. parasomnias

62. Enlarged cerebral ventricles in schizophrenia are associated with:

A. prominent positive symptoms (hallucinations, delusions, etc.)
B. poor premorbid functioning
C. good response to neuroleptics
D. prominent negative symptoms (social withdrawal, abulia, anhedonia, etc.)
E. B and D

63. A patient having a panic attack can experience:

A. palpitations
B. chest pain
C. hand and perioral paresthesias
D. syncope
E. A, B and C

64. A 23-year-old morbidly obese man is admitted to orthopedics with multiple fractures following a car accident during rush-hour traffic, after he fell asleep at the wheel. He reports having frequent uncontrollable 'sleep attacks', more commonly in the afternoon, occurring several times a day. He complains that his night sleep is frequently interrupted and is not restful. His clinical symptoms may be best explained by:

A. narcolepsy
B. primary hypersomnia
C. breathing-related sleep disorder
D. circadian rhythm sleep disorder
E. A and C

65. A 29-year-old woman presents to your office stating that she is concerned that her excessive exposure to sunlight may lead to wrinkles. She asks you whether or not sun exposure causes wrinkles and is interested in the research done in this area. You explain to her that causality can be determined by:

A. observational studies
B. case-control studies
C. cross-sectional studies
D. crossover studies
E. none of the above

66. A 24-year-old woman comes to your office complaining of having frequent urinary tract infections (UTIs). You postulate that ingesting large quantities of cranberry juice will decrease the number of UTIs. If your hypothesis is correct, but you (wrongly) reject it, this is called:

A. type II error
B. β error
C. type I error
D. confounding
E. none of the above

67. The type of error in the question above is equivalent to:

A. the p value
B. $(1 - p)$
C. the power
D. $(p + 1)/2$
E. none of the above

68. You are designing a study that will examine the association between facial fractures and motor vehicle accidents. You are interested in whether the use of an air bag has a substantial impact on the type or number of fractures that result from the accident. One of the issues that you are concerned about in study design is that your study will be sufficiently powered to address this question. Power is equivalent to:

A. $(1 - \alpha)$
B. β
C. $(1 - \beta)$
D. $(1 - p)$
E. none of the above

69. CSF studies in patients with suicidal behavior have shown most consistently:

A. decreased levels of 5-hydroxy-indoleacetic acid (5-HIAA)
B. decreased levels of HVA
C. decreased levels of glucose
D. decreased levels of MHPG
E. no difference between patients and controls

70. Decreased latency to REM sleep periods is associated with:

A. chronic benzodiazepine use
B. sleep deprivation
C. acute alcohol consumption
D. a major depressive episode

71. An anxious married couple come your office. The wife has a family history of Duchenne muscular dystrophy. On further questioning she tells you that two of her uncles died before their teens and a younger brother died in a car accident at the age of 6 months. They have recently learned that they are expecting their first baby and are concerned that their baby may be affected with Duchenne muscular dystrophy. Which of the following statements is correct regarding the inheritance of Duchenne muscular dystrophy?

A. Duchenne muscular dystrophy is not inherited
B. only males are carriers but both males and females are affected
C. only females are carriers but only males are affected
D. of the offspring of an affected female, 50% of females will be carriers and 50% of males will be affected
E. all of her children will be affected irrespective of the sex

72. A 55-year-old female is discovered during a hemicolectomy for a right-sided tubulovillous colonic adenocarcinoma to have a type I choledochal cyst, with dilation of most of the common bile duct up until 1 cm proximal to where the CBD enters the pancreas. She is known to have a history of recurrent pancreatitis that is thought to be related to her history of alcohol consumption. It is decided at the time to speak with the patient's husband and obtain consent to resect the cyst. Consent is obtained and the cyst is resected and a Roux-en-Y hepaticojejunostomy is performed. Which of the following is NOT a common long-term complication of allowing a choledochal cyst to remain in this patient?

A. pancreatitis
B. progression to carcinoma
C. cholangitis
D. erosion into portal vein

73. The likely effect of a dopamine infusion at 5 µg/kg/min is:

A. peripheral vasoconstriction and marked tachycardia
B. systemic and renal vasoconstriction
C. renal blood vessel dilation and marked peripheral vasoconstriction
D. increased cardiac output and a small increase in systemic vascular resistance
E. systemic vasodilatation and fall in blood pressure

Clinical examination revision questions

74–83. For each of the diseases listed below select the associated physical signs:

74. Tension pneumothorax

75. Asthma

76. Pneumonia

77. Pleural effusion

78. Atelectasis with bronchial obstruction

79. Pulmonary fibrosis

80. Pneumothorax

81. Emphysema

82. Left-sided heart failure

83. Normal chest

A. trachea central, stony dullness to percussion, a small area of bronchial breathing
B. trachea shifted away from the affected sight, hyperresonance to percussion
C. trachea central, hyperresonance to percussion and decreased breath sounds
D. trachea central, dullness to percussion, crackles and bronchial breathing
E. trachea central, polyphonic wheeze
F. trachea shifted to side of the lesion, decreased breath sounds, dull to percussion
G. trachea central, breath sounds vesicular, resonant to percussion
H. trachea central, cyanosis, finger clubbing, resonant to percussion, crackles
I. trachea central, stony dullness in the left base, vocal fremitus, wheeze, crackles at bases
J. trachea central, hyperinflated chest, hyperresonance to percussion and loss of cardiac dullness

84–93. Match the cardiac lesion with the clinical findings given below:

84. Aortic stenosis

85. Aortic incompetence

86. Mitral stenosis

87. Mitral incompetence

88. Ventricular septal defect

89. Atrial septal defect

90. Patent ductus arteriosus

91. Tricuspid incompetence

92. Aortic sclerosis

93. Pulmonic stenosis

A. soft S2, midsystolic murmur at the second right interspace radiating to the neck
B. soft S1, pansystolic murmur radiating to the axilla
C. widely fixed split S2 and midsystolic murmur
D. normal heart sounds, harsh pancycle murmur
E. normal S1 and S2, midsystolic murmur radiating to the neck
F. normal heart sounds, early diastolic murmur at the left sternal edge
G. normal heart sounds, pansystolic murmur at the left sternal edge
H. split S2, loud midsystolic murmur, at left midclavicle
I. normal S1 and S2, pansystolic murmur at apex and all over the chest
J. loud S1, middiastolic murmur at apex

TEST FOUR: ANSWERS

1. Answer: E

The history of recent drug ingestion and the examination findings of 'target' lesions with mucosal involvement makes Stevens–Johnson syndrome the likely diagnosis. Stevens–Johnson syndrome is a variant of erythema multiforme where there is mucosal membrane and eye involvement. Other causes of erythema multiforme and Stevens–Johnson syndrome include viral and bacterial infections.

Reference: MacKie, p. 255

2. Answer: A

This boy has the characteristic facial appearance of tuberous sclerosis. The slide shows multiple facial fibromata. The history of mental retardation and epilepsy further supports this diagnosis.

Reference: MacKie, p. 287

3. Answer: A

The lesion shown has the characteristic appearance of a basal cell papilloma. Histologically, there is benign proliferation of epidermal keratinocytes and these lesions become commoner with increasing age. They have a superficial 'stuck on' appearance which helps with the clinical diagnosis. If any doubts exist about these lesions, a biopsy should be done. Acceptable treatment is curettage and diathermy.

Reference: MacKie, p. 339

4A. Answer: B

The skin of the hands is tightly bound, smooth and shiny. There are also atrophic changes of the skin and nails of the right hand. The most likely diagnosis is scleroderma. Biopsy of the skin in scleroderma shows a reduction in the thickness of the dermis. Endarteritis and inflammatory changes are found around blood vessels.

Reference: MacKie, pp. 175–7

4B. Answer: E

Many organ systems are involved in scleroderma. Cardiovascular, pulmonary renal, gastrointestinal endocrine/exocrine function, musculoskeletal and skin complications are all recognized complications. However, infertility is not a recognized complication.

Reference: Kelley, p. 1150

5. Answer: C

The pattern of joint involvement in this patient is consistent with rheumatoid arthritis. Metacarpophalangeal and proximal interphalangeal joints are involved. The wrists and knees are also affected in rheumatoid arthritis. However, joint involvement is only one of the criteria required to make a diagnosis of rheumatoid arthritis. Four or more of the following must be satisfied for at least 6 weeks to confirm a diagnosis of rheumatoid arthritis. These are: morning stiffness, arthritis of three or more joint areas, arthritis of the hands, symmetric arthritis, rheumatoid nodules, rheumatoid factor and radiographic changes.

Reference: Kelley, p. 1114

6A. Answer: B

There are multiple areas of cutaneous depigmentation. Cutaneous depigmentation occurs with both leprosy and vitiligo. However, in leprosy the depigmented areas are anesthetic. Histologically there is loss of melanocytes in the epidermis.

Reference: MacKie, pp. 128, 213

6B. Answer: E

Vitiligo is associated with other autoimmune diseases such as Graves disease, Hashimoto thyroiditis, diabetes mellitus, pernicious anemia, hypoparathyroidism and premature ovarian failure.

Reference: MacKie, p. 213

7. Answer: A

This is Battle's sign. Together with the raccoon sign (periorbital ecchymosis) this suggests, but does not confirm, fracture of the base of the skull.

Reference: Marshall and Mayer, p. 125

8. Answer: D

This woman has a cataract in her right eye. Steroids, radiation, aging and chronic irritation all cause cataracts. Digoxin has not been associated with cataracts.

Reference: Bates, p. 175

9A. Answer: E

The lesion shown is pyoderma gangrenosum, which is not associated with Lyme disease. The lesions of pyoderma gangrenosum are caused by underlying vasculitis. Myeloma may also cause pyoderma gangrenosum.

Reference: MacKie, p. 201

9B. Answer: B

Inflammatory bowel disease is a concern in this patient. In view of the diarrhea and rectal bleeding, CBC and electrolytes to exclude electrolyte disturbance and anemia is appropriate in the first instance. The ESR is useful for monitoring disease activity. Colonoscopy and biopsy will be required to make the ultimate diagnosis. An alternative to colonoscopy is flexible sigmoidoscopy and barium enema. Stool cultures with microscopy to exclude an infectious cause for the symptoms are also important, although infections do not cause pyoderma gangrenosum. A barium meal and gastro-scopy have no place in the initial investigations.

Reference: Kelley, p. 740

10.   Answer: A

There is pitting of the nails and onycholysis. These changes are seen in a proportion of patients with longstanding psoriasis. Nail discoloration may also occur.

Reference: MacKie, pp. 45–6

11.   Answer: E

The history and examination and the facial features make acromegaly the likely diagnosis. Old photographs are valu-able to see serial changes in the facial appearance. An oral glucose tolerance test with growth hormone measurements helps to make the diagnosis. (There is poor or no suppression of growth hormone after glucose administration.) A CT or MRI scan to rule out pituitary tumor is required. Pituitary tumors cause compression of the chiasm and produce visual field defects. Features of acromegaly include large hands and feet, prognathism, coarsening of facial features, proximal muscle weakness, carpal tunnel syndrome, cardiomyopathy, goitre and impotence. Visual evoked potentials are helpful in the diagnosis of demyelinating diseases.

Reference: Kelley, p. 2195

12.   Answer: A

The lesion shown is granuloma annulare. These are erythe-matous raised lesions with well demarcated borders. They occur in children and adults. In adults granuloma annulare may be associated with diabetes.

Reference: MacKie, pp. 275–6

13A. Answer: A

This patient has ankylosing spondylitis. The patient has the typical 'question mark' posture with loss of lumbar lordosis, kyphosis and hyperextension of the neck. (The incidental finding on the angiogram shows ankylosis of the vertebral spine (bamboo spine)).

Reference: Kelley, pp. 1126–30

13B. Answer: E

Ankylosing spondylitis is not associated with renal artery or vein thrombosis. Other features include amyloidosis, iritis and periostitis.

Reference: Kelley, pp. 1126–30

14A. Answer: A

There are multiple plaques of psoriasis on the trunk and arm. The pattern formed by these plaques, as seen in this patient, is sometimes referred to as geographical psoriasis.

Reference: MacKie, p. 46

14B. Answer: D

Steroids can be used in the treatment of psoriasis. Lithium, antimalarials and β-blockers can exacerbate psoriasis.

Reference: MacKie, p. 46

15.   Answer: B

The history of hypotension, hyperkalemia and hyponatremia taken together with dark palmar creases and dark mucus membranes makes adrenocortical deficiency the likely diag-nosis. Pituitary output of melanocyte-stimulating hormone and ACTH is increased. Both of these stimulate melanogenesis.

Reference: MacKie, p. 216

16.   Answer: B

There is involvement of the distal interphalangeal joints, with Heberden's nodes. These findings are consistent with osteoarthritis.

Reference: Rudy and Kurowski, p. 420

17.   Answer: C

Diabetes does not cause cirrhosis but does cause fatty changes in the liver. Other causes of cirrhosis include hepatitis B and C infection and α-1-antitrypsin deficiency.

Reference: Kelley, pp. 818–53

18.   Answer: A

Ehlers–Danlos syndrome is a genetically inherited disorder. There is a defect in dermal collagen. Clinical features include fragile and hyperelastic skin. The joints have lax capsules and are hyperextendable and undergo sublaxation easily. Blood vessels may also be involved. Pseudoxanthoma elasticum is a disorder of elastic tissue but hyperextendable joints is not a typical feature.

Reference: MacKie, pp. 184–6

19.   Answer: A

This woman has a right carotid dissection. She has Horner syndrome on the right and left hemiparesis. Causes of dissect-ion include idiopathic, trauma, fibromuscular dysplasia and other collagen vascular disorders.

Reference: MacKie, pp. 184–6; Samuels and Feske, p. 188

20. Answer: A

A number of gouty tophi are seen on the fingers. Therefore the most likely diagnosis is chronic tophaceous gout. Chronic gout can lead to gross joint destruction resulting in a mutilated appearance of the hand called arthritis mutilans.

Reference: Kelley, p. 1134

21. Answer: B

There is complete paralysis of the left side of the face. Since there is both upper and lower facial involvement, a peripheral facial nerve lesion is the most likely diagnosis.

Reference: Samuels and Feske, pp. 74–5

22. Answer: B

The right hypoglossal nerve is involved. The tongue deviates to the side of the lesion.

Reference: Lindsay et al., p. 18

23. Answer: A

This patient has hereditary hemorrhagic telangectasia, also called Rendu–Osler–Weber syndrome. There are telang-ectasias of the tongue. They also occur in the conjunctivae, ears, skin, face, lung, GI tract and nasopharynx. Prolonged epistaxis is common and GI bleeding can be life-threatening. All the others listed can also cause GI bleeding.

Reference: Kelley, p. 874

24. Answer: A

This man has ptosis and the eyeball is externally and inferiorly rotated (down and out). This is a lesion of the third cranial nerve. The oculomotor nerve carries sympathetic fibers that supply the levator palpebral superioris. The parasympathetic fibers travel on the outside of the nerve. A complete third nerve palsy will have a dilated pupil. The pupil is not well seen in this photograph.

Reference: Samuels and Feske, p. 53

25. Answer: C

This is pemphigus vulgaris, an autoimmune disease that gives rise to erosions and blisters of the skin and mucosa. The lesions are not itchy but can be very painful. Lateral pressure of the skin appears to result in the epidermis passing over the dermis, Nikolsky's sign. These lesions may sponta-neously remit. Oral steroids may shorten the duration and severity of the episodes and are the usual treatment.

Reference: MacKie, pp. 247–9

26. Answer: E

This is shingles caused by the chickenpox virus and is primarily a disease of adult life and old age. In the young it should alert the physician to the possibility of underlying immunosuppression. Spontaneous resolution occurs in 7–10 days but treatment with aciclovir reduces the duration and severity of the disease.

Reference: MacKie, p. 139

27. Answer: A

Erythema ab igne is caused by heat applied to the affected area. The shins and the lower back are commonly affected areas. The shins are affected because the patients sit close to the heating device, while lesions on the lower back are commonly due to hot water bottles. Pretibial myxedema is associated with hyperthryoidism. Necrobiosis lipoidica and granuloma annulare are associated with diabetes.

28. Answer: A

The lesions shown are necrobiosis lipoidica which are assoc-iated with diabetes mellitus. However, these lesions may predate the appearance of diabetes by many years. The lesions are shiny red or yellow plaques which may ulcerate and heal slowly. The individual lesions have marked telangectasis. Good diabetic control does not affect the severity of these lesions.

Reference: MacKie, pp. 274–5

29. Answer: E

The diagnosis is TB. The X-ray shows cavitating lesions in both apices. The X-ray appearance, together with the history, makes TB the likely diagnosis. Underlying immunosuppression should be excluded in this young patient.

Reference: Kelley, pp. 1995–9

30. Answer: C

This is Cullen's sign. It is caused by dissection of blood-tinged ascites along the fascial planes to subcutaneous tissues. (Grey Turner's sign is discoloration at the flanks associated with acute pancreatitis and is caused by a similar mechanism.)

Reference: Kelley, p. 799

31. Answer: E

Neurofibromatosis is transmitted by autosomal dominant inheritance. Optic and acoustic neuromas and peripheral nerve lesions are common. This is a neurocutaneous disorder associated with café au lait spots of the skin and neuro-fibromas of the skin and viscera.

Reference: MacKie, p. 285; Kelley, p. 281

32. Answer: E

The history strongly suggests meningeal irritation. The petechial rash makes the diagnosis of meningococcal menin-gitis most likely. Immediate treatment with ampicillin and ceftriaxone should be started and should not be delayed for LP. The antibiotics can be changed once the sensitivities are known.

Reference: Samuels and Feske, p. 369

33. Answer: A

This is rhinophyma which is a severe chronic form of rosacea. Rhinophyma particularly affects males. Rosacea is characterized by dilation of the vessels in the papillary dermis and sebaceous gland hyperplasia. Removal or shaving of the excessive soft tissue followed by plastic surgery is a treatment option for this disfiguring condition.

Reference: MacKie, pp. 81–2

34. Answer: C

The transverse lines are Beau lines and are associated with temporary arrest and then regrowth of the nail following prolonged serious illness. The condition is self-limiting.

Reference: MacKie, p. 237

35. Answer: C

This is grade IV hypertensive retinopathy. The increased blood pressure in association with heart failure, renal failure and encephalopathy make malignant hypertension the likely diagnosis. Features of hypertensive retinopathy include 'copper wiring', arteriovenous nipping, hard exudates (leakage from arteries), macular edema, retinal hemorrhages and papilledema. Grade I is the mildest and grade IV the most severe.

Reference: Kelley, p. 179

36. Answer: A

The patchy dark pigmentation seen in the retina makes retinitis pigmentosa the likely diagnosis.

37. Answer: C

Clubbing is a triad of loss of the angle between the nail and nail bed, fluctuant nail bed and spooning of the fingers. It is not associated with COPD. Other causes include supportive lung disease and cyanotic heart disease.

Reference: MacKie, p. 238

38. Answer: A

Ulnar nerve entrapment is the likely cause of the changes shown. The elbow is the most common site for this to occur.

Reference: Samuels and Feske, p. 1205

39. Answer: A

The angiogram shows bilateral renal artery stenosis. The aorta is ragged, suggesting marked atherosclerosis, which is also probably affecting the coronary arteries. Renal artery stenosis is an etiological factor for hypertension. He is particularly at risk of developing renal failure from renal hypoperfusion if given ACE inhibitors or angiotensin receptor antagonists. Bilateral renal artery stenosis is a contraindication for ACE inhibitors and angiotensin receptor antagonists.

Reference: Kelley, p. 177

40. Answer: D

This is orf, which is caused by a pox virus and is contracted by contact with sheep. The lesion expands rapidly and develops a necrotic center and is associated with systemic symptoms.

There may also be lymphadenopathy and lymphangitis. However, the lesion resolves spontaneously and one attack usually confers immunity.

Reference: MacKie, p. 135

41. Answer: B

This man has genital herpes, which is caused by herpes type II virus. This is a sexually transmitted disease. Treatment with antivirals may reduce the frequency and severity of the recurrent attacks.

Reference: Kelley, pp. 1762–4

42. Answer: A

The slide shows an hyphema, blood in the anterior chamber of the eye. The usual causes of this include trauma to the eye but it may co-exist with other serious conditions such as lens dislocation, ruptured globe and lens detachment.

Reference: Kelley, p. 256

43. Answer: E

Macroglossia is not a sign of infective endocarditis. Other features include: Osler nodes (painful lesions found on the pads of the fingers and toes), Janeway lesions (vasculitis of the skin) and clubbing.

Reference: Kelley, p. 1588

44. Answer: A

Careful examination of the X-ray shows the characteristic 'hair on ends' appearance of the skull. In thalassemia there is massive marrow hyperplasia, especially around the maxillary sinus, giving the 'chipmunk' appearance of the face.

Reference: Kelley, p. 1439

45. Answer: A

The likely diagnosis is melanoma. The lesion is raised, irregular and pigmented in a patient who works outdoors and is therefore exposed to the sun. The raised ulcerated nodule is a bad prognostic sign. An excision biopsy is needed to make the diagnosis and to assess the degree of spread.

Reference: MacKie, pp. 326–32

46. Answer: A

A patchy pneumonia radiating out from the hili in an immunocompromised patient make *Pneumocystis* pneumonia the likely diagnosis. Other pneumonias can also do this.

Reference: Kelley, pp. 1816–19

47. Answer: D

Radio-opaque lines are seen at the metaphyseal plates; these are leadlines. Lead is preferentially deposited at the metaphyseal plate in children. The increasing weakness and somnolence in this patient is probably due to lead encephalopathy.

Reference: Kelley, p. 2404

48.   Answer: D

Amiodarone is not associated with hirsutism or hypertrichosis. This patient developed hypertrichosis from cyclosporine therapy. Androgen excess can also cause hirsutism and is associated with virilization.

Reference: Kelley, p. 2149

49.   Answer: B

The combination of arthritis, urethritis and iritis fits with the triad of Reiter syndrome. Pustular lesions on the soles of the feet and the arthritis can make distinguishing Reiter syndrome from psoriasis difficult. Reiter syndrome is a seronegative arthropathy. Other features include sacroiliitis, keratoderma blennorrhagicum, painless mouth ulcers, circinate balanitis and entesopathy (plantar fascitis, achilles tendinitis). Reiter syndrome typically begins 2–4 weeks following a diarrheal illness or venereal exposure. Recovery takes several months.

Reference: Kelley, p. 1128

50.   Answer: D

Both the barium study and the pathology specimen show small bowel diverticulosis. The small bowel can be distinguished from adjacent areas by the presence of plicae circulares that are clearly visible on the barium study. Small bowel diverticulosis is rare but associated with malabsorption in the small bowel due to bacterial overgrowth (the accident was unrelated).

51.   Answer: E

Diabetes is not associated with atopic dermatitis. Hay fever, asthma, food intolerance and viral infections such as molluscum contagiosum and herpes are all associated. The itchy lesions commonly affect the flexural surfaces.

Reference: MacKie, pp. 91–100

52.   Answer: A

This is the characteristic 'butterfly' rash of systemic lupus erythematosus and may be provoked by sunlight and a variety of drugs including sulfonamides, penicillin, oral contraceptives, isoniazid, griseofulvin, hydralazine and procainamide.

Reference: MacKie, pp. 168–9

53.   Answer: B

This is lichen planus. This cutaneous disorder comprises intensely itchy flat-topped papules on the wrists and lower legs. The mucus membranes are also affected as shown. Spontaneous resolution takes months to years. Antihistamines, intralesional and systemic steroids have been tried with limited success. The etiology is unknown but gold, diuretics and antimalarials can trigger lichen planus.

Reference: MacKie, pp. 59–60

54.   Answer: A

This is condyloma acuminatum, caused by the human papilloma virus. It is transmitted by sexual contact although vertical transmission is recognized. It spontaneously regresses over months to years.

Reference: Kelley, p. 1788

55.   Answer: E

Gynecomastia, excess of breast tissue, is not associated with ranitidine. Other associations include Klinefelter syndrome, Kallmann disease, estrogens, marijuana, spironolactone, hyperthyroidism and testosterone.

Reference: Kelley, p. 2159

56.   Answer: C

Gastroschisis and omphalocele are two relatively common congenital malformations that pediatric surgeons are faced with. Gastroschisis is a ventral abdominal wall defect that is believed to result from abnormal epidermal development. The defect is usually to the right of the midline, and there is typically no membrane sac that envelops the herniated viscera. Herniated viscera may be coated with a fibrinous coating. There is a propensity for significant loss of heat and fluid from the defect, and treatment is emergent; definitive treatment involves reduction of the eviscerated organs and repair of the abdominal wall defect. A staged reduction can be performed using a silo. Omphaloceles involve a wall defect at the umbilicus. The herniated viscera are bound by a sac consisting of an inner layer of peritoneum and an external layer of amnion. Management of omphaloceles is similar to that of gastroschisis, but is generally considered to be less emergent.

Reference: Sabiston, pp. 1247–8

57.   Answer: A

Approximately 2500 liver transplants are performed each year for a variety of indications, most commonly for primary cholestatic liver disease, cirrhosis (usually alcoholic, due to hepatitis B/C, or autoimmune), fulminant hepatic failure, and metabolic disorders. Patients with primary cholestatic disease (PBC, PSC) have 5-year survivals of approximately 80%. Success of the procedure depends on many factors, notably the timing of the procedure along the progression of the disease. Initial reluctance to transplant patients with cirrhosis due to alcoholism has waned recently, and several studies have established a recidivism rate in the 11–12% range, not high enough to warrant exclusion based on this criterion alone. A 6-month period of abstinence is generally required prior to the procedure, however. Procured livers have a relatively long preservation time; using the University of Wisconsin (UW) solution, livers have been preserved for up to 3 days. The goal of the transplant team, obviously, is to transplant the organ as quickly as possible. It is much more difficult to preserve the heart, which can only be preserved for approximately 4 hours prior to transplantation. For children with biliary atresia, a partial liver transplant is usually not the procedure of choice. A Kasai portoenterostomy, or some variation thereof, is generally performed. Between 30 and 40% of these patients will not require a liver transplant, and a significant body of them can delay transplant until years later, when the procedure is less technically difficult and outcomes are improved.

Reference: Sabiston, pp. 461–3

58. Answer: D

The postoperative course following liver transplantation is fraught with complications. Most immediately, primary nonfunction occurs in 5–10% of cases, necessitating an almost immediate lifesaving retransplantation. Primary nonfunction is defined as that occurring within 96 hours of the transplant, and in the presence of a functioning portal vein and hepatic artery. Hepatic artery thrombosis is an important complication to be vigilant against, as the sole blood supply of the transplanted common bile duct is from this vessel. When stricture of the common bile duct occurs (usually at the site of anastomosis), the hepatic artery is often implicated. While technical flaws are a factor in many cases of hepatic artery thrombosis, more often than not no flaw is discovered. The newly transplanted liver is often slow to produce anticoagulant proteins and there is often a period of postoperative hypercoagulability that is probably a causative factor. Portal vein thrombosis is a relatively rare occurrence, seen in only 1–2% of cases.

Reference: Greenfield, p. 592

59. Answer: A

Early menarche, family history, obesity and late first pregnancy are all risk factors for breast cancer. Early menopause is not considered a risk factor. The reason for the increased risk is not known but longer duration of exposure to estrogens may be one explanation.

Reference: Kelley, p. 1337

60. Answer: A

Doppler ultrasound and venograms are helpful in the diagnosis of deep venous thrombosis. Radioactive fibrinogen scanning can also help in the diagnosis but is not routinely used in clinical practice. Clinical diagnosis is difficult and often only detects 50% of confirmed deep venous thrombosis. Emboli are more likely to originate from the thigh veins than the calf veins. The incidence of pulmonary emboli is underestimated.

Reference: Rudy and Kurowski, pp. 109–16

61. Answer: D

Acute alcohol administration causes REM sleep suppression in the first half of the night followed by a rebound increase of REM sleep with multiple arousals in the second half.

Alcohol intoxication reduces respiratory drive and can cause episodes of apnea during slow sleep. Parasomnias are not associated with acute alcohol intoxication.

Reference: Hales and Yudofsky, p. 791

62. Answer: E

Cerebral ventricular enlargement is the most consistently replicated biological finding in schizophrenia, but sulcal enlargement and cerebellar atrophy have also been reported. There is substantial evidence to suggest that ventricular enlargement is associated with poor premorbid functioning, negative symptoms, poor response to treatment and cognitive impairment. Computer tomographic abnormalities occur in up to 40% of schizophrenics, although there is a predominant male effect and the changes are not specific for this pathologic entity.

Reference: Hales and Yudofsky, p. 415

63. Answer: E

The DSM–IV defines a panic attack as a discrete period of intense fear or discomfort, in which at least four symptoms from a list develop abruptly and reach a peak within 10 minutes. The symptoms include palpitations, diaphoresis, trembling, dyspnea (or sensation of smothering), feeling of choking, chest pain, nausea or abdominal distress, dizziness, lightheadedness, unsteadiness or faintness, derealization or depersonalization, paresthesias, chills or hot flushes, and fears of losing control, going crazy or dying. Syncope is not a manifestation of a panic attack and should call for a specific workup.

Reference: DSM–IV, pp. 394–5

64. Answer: A

The history of irresistible 'sleep attacks' at different times of the day, and even during normal driving, is suggestive of narcolepsy. The diagnosis of narcolepsy would be supported by the presence of cataplexy, hypnagogic or hypnopompic hallucinations, and sleep paralysis. Patients with primary hypersomnia also have daytime sleepiness which is, however, characteristically less urgent than the sleep attacks of narcolepsy, and unintentional sleep occurs only at periods of low stimulation (e.g. lectures, watching TV, etc.). In these patients the night sleep is prolonged (10–12 hours) and normal in quality. On the other hand, in breathing-related sleep disorder the degree of daytime sleepiness is equal in magnitude to that of individuals with narcolepsy. Breathing-related sleep disorder is distinguished from narcolepsy by a history of loud snoring, breathing pauses that disrupt normal sleep, lengthy and unrefreshing daytime naps and the absence of associated symptoms of narcolepsy. However, the definite diagnosis in this patient may require polysomnographic recording with oxygen saturation monitoring. Circadian rhythm sleep disorder is defined by a persistent or recurrent pattern of sleep disruption that results from a mismatch between the individual's endogenous circadian rhythm, and exogenous demands regarding the timing and duration of sleep (e.g. jet-lag, shift work, etc.).

Reference: DSM–IV, pp. 553–78

65. Answer: E

While these studies demonstrate an association between two factors, they cannot conclusively determine that one causes the other. Therefore, while there are several studies that demonstrate an association between sun exposure and wrinkles, none actually prove that sun exposure causes wrinkles. This is analogous to the tobacco industry's claims that smoking has never been shown to cause lung cancer, only that the two are associated. A randomized controlled trial of smoking versus nonsmoking and the development of lung cancer is clearly not feasible owing to both practical and ethical concerns.

Reference: Hennekens *et al.*, pp. 30–53

66. Answer: C

Type I error is synonymous with α error and type II error is synonymous with β error. This is a case of type I error, where the null hypothesis is true but we wrongly reject it. Type II (β) error is when the null hypothesis is false but we fail to reject it.

Reference: Mould, p. 78

67. Answer: A

The *p* value reflects the likelihood of erroneously rejecting the null hypothesis, and therefore is equivalent to the type I error. The relationship between the power of a study and error will be addressed in the following question.

Reference: Mould, p. 78

68. Answer: C

The power of a study reflects the probability of rejecting the null hypothesis and concluding that there is a statistically significant difference when one truly exists. It is therefore equivalent to $1 - \beta$ (or 1 – the type II error) of a study.

Reference: Mould, p. 78

69. Answer: A

Studies of postmortem brains have demonstrated a high correlation between the tissue levels of the serotonin metabolite 5-HIAA and its CSF levels; thus, the latter have been considered reflective of CNS functioning. Numerous studies have shown that depressed patients who have made suicide attempts have decreased levels of 5-HIAA in CSF, and this may predict the risk of future suicide in as many as 21% of these patients within 1 year. Similar data have been reproduced in alcoholics, schizophrenics and patients with borderline personality disorder, but this change may be absent in patients with bipolar affective disorders.

Reference: Hales and Yudofsky, pp. 1160–1

70. Answer: C

Sleep deprivation from any cause produces daytime sleepiness and other symptoms related to shortened REM latency (sleep paralysis or sleep-related hallucinations). A sleep disturbance is identifiable in 90% of patients with major depression, and is characterized by sleep fragmentation, decreased quantity and altered distribution of δ sleep, reduced REM latency, redistribution of REM sleep into the first part of the night, and increased frequency of eye movements during REM. Acute alcohol administration causes suppression of REM sleep during the first half of the night (i.e. prolongs latency), followed by a rebound increase of REM in the second half of the night with increased arousals. Chronic benzodiazepine use does not significantly change latency to the first REM period.

Reference: Hales and Yudofsky, pp. 787–91; DSM–IV, pp. 565–6

71. Answer: D

Duchenne muscular dystrophy is a devastating neurological condition that exhibits X-linked recessive inheritance. If this woman is a carrier, then 50% of her female offspring will be carriers and 50% of her male offspring will be affected. The abnormal gene product in this condition is reduced amounts of a structural protein called dystrophin.

Reference: Fenichel, pp. 181–3

72. Answer: D

Choledochal cysts are a phenomenon with no clear etiology, but which occur more commonly in males than females. There are five major types of choledochal cyst, each type varying in the manifestation of intrahepatic or extrahepatic ductal dilation (or both). Their presence poses an increased risk for several disorders of the biliary system, and they should be removed whenever encountered. The dilated ductal system often has points of stricture, and diversionary procedures (used in the past) left a 20% likelihood of progression to carcinoma. A complete excision of the cyst and Roux-en-Y hepaticojejunostomy is currently the most widely accepted procedure. Cholangitis and pancreatitis are also known to occur with increased frequency in patients with choledochal cysts. Erosion or fistulization into the portal vein is not a common complication of choledochal cysts.

Reference: Sabiston, pp. 1258–9

73. Answer: D

Dopamine has β-1 and α effects. The effect of dopamine depends on the dose. A dose of 1–2 µg/kg/min of dopamine has a direct effect on dopaminergic receptors to produce cerebral, renal and mesenteric vasodilatation, and urine output may increase. At doses of 2–10 µg/kg/min the β-1 effect causes an increase in cardiac output and partly antagonizes the α effect of vasoconstriction on the peripheral vasculature. At higher doses there is a marked increase in renal mesenteric peripheral arterial and venous vasoconstriction.

Reference: Cummins, p. 8.3

74–83 (see also Table 1).

74. Answer: B
75. Answer: E
76. Answer: D
77. Answer: A
78. Answer: F
79. Answer: H
80. Answer: C
81. Answer: J
82. Answer: I
83. Answer: G

84–93 (see also Table 2).

84. Answer: A
85. Answer: F
86. Answer: J
87. Answer: B
88. Answer: I
89. Answer: C
90. Answer: D
91. Answer: G
92. Answer: E
93. Answer: H

Table 1 Diseases and their physical signs. Refer to answers 74–83

	Trachea	Percussion	Vocal resonance/ fremitus	Breath sounds	Added sounds
Tension pneumothorax	away	hyperresonant	decreased	decreased	none
Asthma	central	hyperresonant	normal	decreased	wheeze
Pneumonia	central	dull	increased	bronchial	crackles
Pleural effusion	central	stony dull	decreased	decreased	none
Atelectasis	same side	dull	decreased	decreased	none
Pulmonary fibrosis	central	resonant	normal	vesicular	crackles
Pneumothorax	central	hyperresonant	decreased	decreased	none
Emphysema	central	hyperresonant	decreased	vesicular	none
Left heart failure	central	resonant	normal	vesicular	crackles
Normal chest	central	resonant	normal	vesicular	none

Table 2 Cardiac lesions and their associated clinical findings (simplified). Refer to answers 84–93

	Heart sounds	Murmur	Location	Radiation	Apex
Aortic stenosis	soft S2	midsystolic	second right interspace	neck	undisplaced
Aortic incompetence	normal S1 and S2	early diastolic	left sternal border	apex	displaced
Mitral stenosis	loud S1	middiastolic	apex	none	undisplaced
Mitral incompetence	soft S1, loud S3	pansystolic	apex	axilla	displaced
VSD	normal S1 and S2	harsh pansystolic	apex and third/fourth/ fifth interspace	all over the chest	undisplaced
ASD	wide fixed splitting S2	midsystolic	second left interspace	none	undisplaced
PDA	normal S1 and S2	continuous	second left interspace	left clavicle	undisplaced
Tricuspid incompetence	normal S1 and S2	pansystolic	left sternum	left mid-clavicle	undisplaced
Aortic sclerosis	normal S1 and S2	midsystolic	apex	neck	undisplaced
Pulmonic stenosis	widely split S2	midsystolic	left mid-clavicle	left shoulder	undisplaced

Reference: Bates, pp. 300–10; VSD, ventricular septal defect; ASD, atrial septal defect; PDA, patent ductus arteriosus

REFERENCES

Adams RD, Victor M, Ropper AH. *Adams' and Victor's Principles of Neurology.* New York: McGraw Hill, 1997

American Psychiatric Association. *Diagnostic and Statistical Manual of Mental Disorders* (4th edn.) (DSM–IV). Washington, DC: American Psychiatric Press, 1994

Baldor RA, Humphreys TR. Malignant melanoma. *Hosp Physician* 1998;34:27–37

Bates B. *Guide to Physical Examination and History Taking.* Philadelphia: Lippincott, 1987

Bernard GR, Artigas A, Brigham KL, *et al.* The American–European Consensus Conference on ARDS: definitions, mechanisms, relevant outcomes and clinical trial coordination. *Am Rev Respir Crit Care Med* 1994;149: 818–24

Berson FG. *Basic Ophthalmology for Medical Students and Primary Care Residents.* San Francisco: American Academy of Ophthalmology, 1993

Bradley WG, Daroff RB, Fenichel GM, Marsden D. *Neurology in Clinical Practice: Volume 1* (3rd edn.). Boston: Butterworth–Heinemann, 2000

Cullom RD, Chang B. *The Wills Eye Manual – Office and Emergency Room Diagnosis and Treatment of Eye Disease* (2nd edn.). Philadelphia: J. B. Lippincott Company, 1994

Cummins RO. *Advanced Cardiac Life Support.* Dallas: American Heart Association, 1997

David TE. Surgery of the aortic valve. *Curr Prob Surg* 1999;36:426–501

Dinubile MJ. Surgery in active endocarditis. *Ann Intern Med* 1982;96:650–9

Dornbrand L, Hoole AJ, Fletcher RH. *Manual of Clinical Problems in Adult Ambulatory Care* (3rd edn.). Philadelphia: Lippincott-Raven, 1997

Durand JM, Burtey S. Glomerulonephritis. *Lancet* 1999;353:1509–15

Ewald GA, McKenzie CR. *Manual of Medical Therapeutics* (28th edn.). Boston: Little, Brown and Co., 1997

Executive summary of the clinical guidelines on the identification, evaluation and treatment of overweight and obesity in adults. *Arch Intern Med* 1998;158:1855–67

Fauci AS, Braunwald E, Isselbacher KJ, *et al. Harrison's Principles of Internal Medicine* (14th edn.). New York: McGraw Hill, 1998

Fenichel GM. *Clinical Pediatric Neurology, A Signs and Symptoms Approach* (3rd edn.). Philadelphia: W. B. Saunders Co., 1997

Friedman NJ, Pineda R, Kaiser P. *The Massachusetts Eye and Ear Infirmary Illustrated Manual of Ophthalmology.* Philadelphia: W. B. Saunders Co., 1998

Gertz MA, Lacy MQ, Dispenzieri A. Amyloidosis: recognition, confirmation, prognosis and therapy. *Mayo Clin Proc* 1999;74:490–5

Gilbert DN, Sande MA, Moellering RC. *The Sanford Guide to Antimicrobial Therapy.* Viena, VA: Antimicrobial Therapy, Inc., 1999

Gold MS. *General Surgery Board Review* (3rd edn.). New York: Lippincott-Raven, 1999

Greenberg A, Cheung AK, Falk RJ, Coffman TM. *Primer on Kidney Diseases* (2nd edn.). New York: Academic Press, 1998

Greenfield LJ. *Surgery: Scientific Principles and Practice* (2nd edn.). Philadelphia: Lippincott-Raven, 1997

Guillem JG, Smith AJ, Calle JP, Ruo L. Gastrointestinal polyposis syndromes. *Curr Prob Surg* 1999;36:217–323

Hales RE, Yudofsky SC. *The American Psychiatric Press Synopsis of Psychiatry* (3rd edn.). New York: American Psychiatric Press, 1996

Hampton JR. *The ECG in Practice* (2nd edn.). New York: Churchill Livingstone, 1994

Hardman JG, Limbird LE. *Goodman and Gilman's The Pharmacological Basis of Therapeutics* (9th edn.). New York: McGraw Hill, 1996

Hennekens CH, Buring JE, Mayrent SL. *Epidemiology in Medicine.* Boston: Little, Brown and Co., 1997

Hortobagyi GN. Treatment of breast cancer. *N Engl J Med* 1998;339:974–84

Hull D, Johnston DI. *Essential Pediatrics* (3rd edn.). London: Churchill Livingstone, 1993

Ivatury RR, Diebel L, Porter JM, Simon RJ. Intra-abdominal hypertension and the abdominal compartment syndrome. *Surg Clin North Am* 1997;77:783–800

Kelley WN. *Textbook of Internal Medicine* (3rd edn.). Philadelphia: Lippincott-Raven, 1997

Knopp RH. Drug treatment of lipid disorders. *N Engl J Med* 1999;341:498–511

Kulke MH, Mayer RJ. Carcinoid tumors. *N Engl J Med* 1999;340:858–68

Lagergren JL, Bergstrom R, Lindgren A, Nyren O. Symptomatic gastroesophageal reflux as a risk factor for esophageal adenocarcinoma. *N Engl J Med* 1999;340: 825–31

Leppik IE. *Contemporary Diagnosis and Management of the Patient with Epilepsy* (4th edn.). Newtown, PA: Handbooks in Health Care, 1998

Light RW. *Pleural Diseases* (3rd edn.). Baltimore: Williams & Wilkins, 1995

Lindsay KW, Bone I, Callander R. *Neurology and Neurosurgery Illustrated* (2nd edn.). London: Churchill Livingstone, 1995

MacKie RM. *Clinical Dermatology: An Illustrated Textbook* (3rd edn.). Oxford: Oxford Medical Publications, 1991

Marino PL. *The ICU Book* (2nd edn.). Baltimore: Williams & Wilkins, 1990

Marshall RS, Mayer SA. *On Call Neurology*. Philadelphia: W. B. Saunders Co., 1997

Mould RF. *Introductory Medical Statistics* (2nd edn.). Bristol: Adam Hilger, 1989

Osborne CK. Tamoxifen in the treatment of breast cancer. *N Engl J Med* 1998;339:1609–18

Oski FA, DeAngelis CD, Feigin RD, *et al. Principles and Practice of Pediatrics* (2nd edn.). Philadelphia: J. B. Lippincott, 1994

Powell JW, Barber-Foss KD. Traumatic brain injury in high school athletes. *J Am Med Assoc* 1999;282:958–63

Rockey DC. Occult gastrointestinal bleeding. *N Engl J Med* 1999;341:38–46

Rosner B. *Fundamentals of Biostatistics*. Belmont, CA: Duxbury Press, 1996

Rudy DR, Kurowski K. *Family Medicine*. Baltimore: Williams & Wilkins, 1997

Sabiston DC Jr. *Textbook of Surgery: the Biological Basis of Modern Surgical Practice* (15th edn.). Philadelphia: W. B. Saunders Co., 1997

Samuels MA, Feske S. *Office Practice of Neurology*. London: Churchill Livingstone, 1996

Schoenfeld A, Levavi H, Hirsch M, *et al.* Transvaginal sonography in postmenopausal women. *J Clin Ultrasound* 1990;18:350–8

Singer AJ, Hollander JE, Quinn JV. Evaluation and management of traumatic lacerations. *N Engl J Med* 1997;337: 1142–8

Schlumberger MJ. Medical progress: papillary and follicular thyroid carcinoma. *N Engl J Med* 1998;338:297–306

Sprigings D, Chambers J, Jeffrey A. *Acute Medicine: A Practical Guide to the Management of Medical Emergencies* (2nd edn.). Oxford/London: Blackwell Science, 1995

Symonds EM. *Essential Obstetrics and Gynaecology* (2nd edn.). London: Churchill Livingstone, 1992

Tierney LM, McPhee SJ, Papadakis MA. *Current Medical Diagnosis and Treatment* (36th edn.). Stamford, CT: Appleton and Lange, 1997

Townes AS. Crystal induced arthritis. In Barker LR, Burton JR, Zieve PD, eds. *Principles of Ambulatory Medicine* (5th edn.). Baltimore: Lippincott, Williams & Wilkins, 1995

Vander JF, Gault JA. *Ophthalmology Secrets*. Philadelphia: Hanley & Belfus, Inc., 1998

Wilson FM. *Practical Ophthalmology – A Manual for Beginning Residents*. San Francisco: American Academy of Ophthalmology, 1996

Winokur G, Clayton PJ. *The Medical Basis of Psychiatry*. Philadelphia: W. B. Saunders Co., 1994

Wright KW. *Textbook of Ophthalmology*. Baltimore: Williams & Wilkins, 1997

Yeo CJ, Cameron JL. Pancreatic cancer. *Curr Prob Surg* 1999;36:59–152

Zitelli BJ, Davis HW. *Atlas of Pediatric Physical Diagnosis* (3rd edn.). St. Louis: Mosby-Wolfe, 1997

T - #0441 - 101024 - C8 - 279/216/8 - PB - 9781850700630 - Gloss Lamination